Prostate

Cancer

From

A to Z

Prostate Cancer

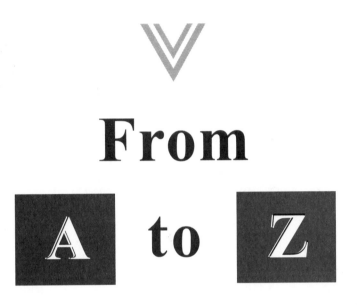

From

A to Z

Kenneth J. Pienta, M.D.
and
Mark A. Moyad, M.P.H.

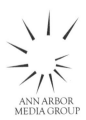

ANN ARBOR
MEDIA GROUP

Prostate Cancer ▶ From A to Z
by Kenneth J. Pienta, M.D. and Mark A. Moyad, M.P.H.

Copyright 2004
Kenneth J. Pienta, M.D. and Mark A. Moyad, M.P.H.

Published by J. W. Edwards, Inc. by special arrangement with
The Ann Arbor Media Group, LLC.
2500 S. State Street
Ann Arbor, Michigan 48104

Cover Design by Steven J. Benedict III
Illustrations by Theodore G. Huff & Associates
Typography by Lor Holland

Printed and bound by Edwards Brothers, Inc., Ann Arbor, MI

ISBN 1-930842-01-5

07 06 05 04   10 9 8 7 6 5 4 3 2 1

CONTENTS

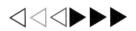

RECENT IMPORTANT MEDICAL RESEARCH

Section

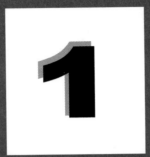

Preventing

Prostate

Cancer

THE PROSTATE PROBLEM

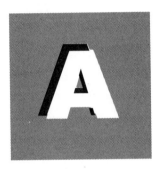

WHAT IS THE NUMBER 1 CANCER DIAGNOSED IN MEN TODAY? COLON? LUNG? SKIN?

NO, IT'S PROSTATE CANCER.

◁ IN FACT ▷

- ▶ Prostate cancer accounts for more than 40% of all the cancers diagnosed in men.
- ▶ Over 200,000 men a year are diagnosed with prostate cancer in the United States.
- ▶ Approximately 1 out of 6 men will be diagnosed with prostate cancer in their lifetime.
- ▶ Every three minutes, someone is diagnosed with prostate cancer.

TABLE 1.—Cancer Incidence

Men		Women	
Type of Incidence	**Percent**	**Type of Incidence**	**Percent**
Prostate	43	Breast	30
Lung	12	Lung	13
Colon & Rectum	8.5	Colon & Rectum	11
Bladder	5	Uterus	6
Non-Hodgkin's Lymphoma	4	Ovary	4.5
Melanoma (skin cancer)	3	Non-Hodgkin's Lymphoma	4
Oral Cavity (mouth & throat)	3	Melanoma (skin ancer)	3
Kidney	2	Bladder	2.5
Leukemia	2	Cervix	2
Stomach	2	Pancreas	2

The point, of course, is that prostate cancer is a fairly common disease.

Prostate cancer is not only increasingly common, it's also serious.

Consider that:

▶ Prostate cancer is the Number 2 cancer killer of men in the United States, second only to lung cancer.

▶ In 1973, 18,830 American men died of prostate cancer. In 2002, almost 32,000 men will die of this disease.

▶ Someone dies of prostate cancer in the United States every 13 minutes.

▶ Deaths due to prostate cancer are also increasing in other parts of the world, such as Australia, Europe, Japan, and Russia.

The growing number of deaths from prostate cancer is not simply the result of a growing population. Over the last 25 years, the prostate cancer death rate—a figure that is

TABLE 2.—Cancer Mortality				
Men			**Women**	
Type of Cancer	**Percent**		**Type of Cancer**	**Percent**
Lung	32		Lung	25
Prostate	14		Breast	16.5
Colon & Rectum	9		Colon & Rectum	10.5
Pancreas	4.5		Pancreas	5.5
Non-Hodgkin's Lymphoma	4		Ovary	5
Leukemia	4		Non-Hodgkin's Lymphoma	4
Esophagus	3		Leukemia	3.5
Stomach	3		Uterus	2
Bladder	2.5		Brain	2
Liver	2.5		Stomach	2

independent of population size—has increased 25%. In other words, a greater percentage of men are dying from prostate cancer than ever before. There is some evidence that the death rate has been declining in the last few years, but until that trend continues for some time, we will be faced with more and more cases of—and deaths from—prostate cancer.

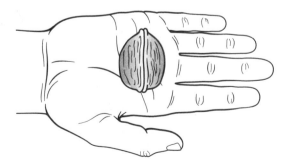

FIGURE A-1.—The prostate gland is approximately the size of a walnut.

Overall, this book is for men, their partners and their families who not only want to know more about prostate cancer in general, but who have localized cancer and are worried about treatment and possible side effects, as well as those who have advanced prostate cancer.

Early detection is the key to fighting this disease. Every man who is thought to have more than 10 years to live should be screened for prostate cancer with a yearly digital rectal exam (DRE) and prostate-specific antigen (PSA) blood test starting at the age of 50. This should start at age 40 if there is a family history or for men of African-American descent.

ESTABLISHED RISK FACTORS: AGE, FAMILY HISTORY, AND RACE

WHERE DOES PROSTATE CANCER COME FROM?

THERE IS NO SIMPLE ANSWER TO THAT QUESTION—NO ONE KNOWS EXACTLY HOW OR WHY MEN GET PROSTATE CANCER. THERE ARE NO SIMPLE GENETIC OR ENVIRONMENTAL CLUES. THERE ARE SEVERAL MAJOR RISK FACTORS ASSOCIATED WITH PROSTATE CANCER IN GENERAL, INCLUDING AGE, RACE, FAMILY HISTORY, AND HORMONE LEVELS. MANY OF THESE FACTORS CANNOT BE CONTROLLED OR AVOIDED, BUT THERE ARE A FEW THAT SOMETHING CAN BE DONE ABOUT. LET'S TAKE A LOOK AT BOTH THE NON-PREVENTABLE AND THE PREVENTABLE RISK FACTORS.

▶ **Age**

The biggest risk factor for prostate cancer is clearly a man's age. In fact, almost 80% of the men diagnosed with prostate cancer are 65 years of age or older. Very few men in their twenties or thirties are diagnosed with prostate cancer. When a group of men in their 50's who had died of other causes was looked at, nearly 1 out of 3 of the men had prostate cancer. By age 70, that climbs to about 70%; by age 80, to just under 80%; and by age 90, to about 90%. The disease is so common in elderly men, who typically have other health problems as well, that doctors often say, "You are more likely to die with prostate cancer than from prostate cancer." That's true, but that saying should not lead anyone to become complacent about the disease. Remember: One of six men will develop prostate cancer that affects his life and approximately one-third of those will develop advanced prostate cancer.

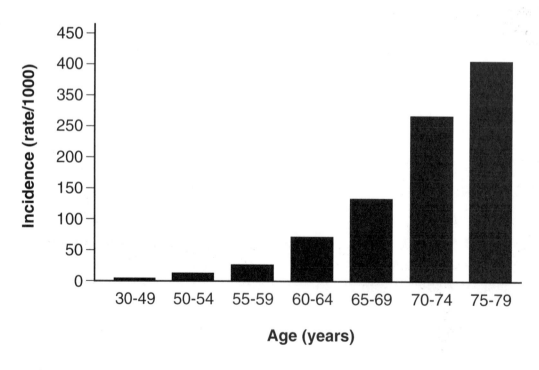

FIGURE B-1.—Age and the development of prostate cancer.

▶ Family History

In the United States, the average man's risk of one day having prostate cancer is between 10% and 15%, and the average man's risk of dying from prostate cancer is 3%. If other family members have had the disease, however, the risk of developing it, and developing it earlier, goes up. If one family member has had prostate cancer, for example, someone's risk is doubled. If two family members have had prostate cancer, the risk becomes two to five times higher. It does not matter whether the person with prostate cancer comes the mother's or the father's side of the family—the risk is still the same.

▶ Race

Ethnic background plays a definite role in prostate-cancer risk. Within the United States, African-Americans are more likely to die of prostate cancer than members of any other race. In fact, African-Americans are about twice as likely to develop prostate cancer than members of any other race. Asians, on the other hand, have the lowest incidence of prostate cancer, while whites fall in between. The reasons for these differences are not yet understood.

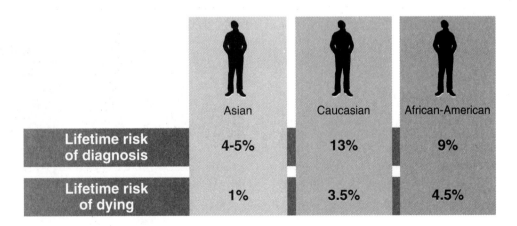

	Asian	Caucasian	African-American
Lifetime risk of diagnosis	4-5%	13%	9%
Lifetime risk of dying	1%	3.5%	4.5%

FIGURE B-2.—Race and the development of prostate cancer.

OTHER POTENTIAL RISK FACTORS

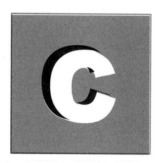

▶ Screening

Every man should have a yearly DRE and PSA blood test to screen for prostate cancer starting at the age of 50, or as early as age 40 if there is a family history or for men of African-American descent. It has recently been demonstrated that screening leads to the detection of more cancers that are localized inside of the prostate. The number of deaths from prostate cancer should decrease as more and more men are cured by primary treatments such as surgery or radiation. Lack of screening increases the chance of being diagnosed with advanced disease.

▶ Environment

While race and location play a role in prostate cancer, when men move from one country to another, they eventually come close to achieving the prostate-cancer risk of their adopted nation. So, if a Chinese man moves from China—where only a small number of men die of prostate cancer—to the United States, his risk of dying from prostate cancer increases to become comparable to that of the average American male. Why this would be so is not well understood. It could be factors in the diet, or even how much sunlight a man is exposed to.

► Sun Exposure

Some scientists suspect that exposure to the sun has an effect on the disease. In the United States, for example, men living in the South have a smaller chance of dying from prostate cancer than men living in the North. The theory is that exposure to ultraviolet (UV) radiation from the sun has a protective effect against prostate cancer—perhaps because UV radiations activates the production of vitamin D in the body, which has been known to have some anticancer effects. This may help explain why prostate cancer death rates are highest in areas with less exposure to the sun's rays, such as Scandinavia and North America. This sun-exposure theory also may help explain why African-American men—even those who live in southern climates—are about twice as likely to develop prostate cancer as anyone else, since their highly pigmented skin absorbs less UV radiation. In addition, this theory may also partially explain why older men of any race are at a higher risk of developing prostate cancer, because aging deceases the body's ability to make vitamin D from sunlight.

► Diet

A diet high in saturated fat (especially animal fat) and low in fiber may increase the risk of prostate cancer. Studies have shown that prostate tumors grow faster in animals fed a high-fat diet. People who live in Asia tend to eat less fat than Americans, which may be a partial explanation for the lower incidence of death from prostate cancer in China and Japan. Beans, lentils, green peas, and even strawberries have been identified as being helpful in lowering risk; however, the strongest data appear to support a balanced diet low in saturated fat (low in calories) and high in fiber, vegetables, and fruit. Not only is this diet good for cancer prevention, it is good for the heart.

► Occupation

Jobs in a number of fields—such as water treatment, aircraft manufacturing, railway transport, utilities, farming, fishing, and forestry—have been associated with prostate cancer risk, but the evidence so far suggests only a slight or possible association. For every study that suggests an increased risk based on a certain occupation, there seems to be another that suggests that this risk does not exist. Slight risks may be related to occupationally-oriented exposure to substances, such as a farmer's use of pesticides. It has been suggested that soldiers exposed to Agent Orange may have an increased risk of getting prostate cancer.

▶ Alcohol

A number of studies seem to indicate that there is little to no risk of getting prostate cancer due to the consumption of alcohol. Some research has suggested that men who drink heavily have a slightly increased risk—heavy drinking meaning 22 to 60 drinks a week or more over many years. On the other hand, another recent study has shown that men consuming 57 drinks or more per week did not have an increased risk of prostate cancer. In any case, men who regularly drink that much are likely to have other health problems more pressing than prostate cancer. When it comes to alcohol and prostate cancer, the old saying holds true: "Everything in moderation." A glass of wine or a beer a day will probably not increase anyone's risk of getting prostate cancer.

▶ Biopsy, TURP, or Other Procedures

Does a biopsy or any other procedure increase the chance of cancer cells getting into the bloodstream and spreading beyond the prostate?" Researchers do not agree on whether a biopsy or transurethral resection of the prostate (TURP), a treatment for benign prostate problems, can spread cancer. Overall, it appears that there is a minimal risk with these procedures, in large part because any cells released into the bloodstream are subject to high pressures and the body's immune system, which can be very effective at destroying a few stray cancer cells. More importantly, a biopsy is still the most accurate way of determining whether or not someone has cancer and how aggressive the cancer is—it is far better to perform the procedure than to simply "guess" about the presence and aggressiveness of cancer based on laboratory tests and other indirect clinical information.

If someone has to have multiple biopsies for any reason, it may be a good idea to wait several weeks between them, which is usually the way such tests are handled. In general, of course, a biopsy should only be done when the presence of cancer is suspected based on other information (such as a physical exam or PSA test). A TURP should only be done on people whose noncancerous problems are not treatable by less invasive means such as natural therapy and medication.

▶ PIN

There are two types of PIN: Low-grade PIN, which used to be called "PIN1," and high-grade PIN, which used to be known as "PIN2" or "PIN3." Only high-grade PIN is associated with an increased possibility of having cancer. The discovery of low-grade PIN does not put someone at a higher risk of having prostate cancer, and clinicians cannot agree on exactly what it looks like. So, many pathologists have stopped trying to identify and report low-grade PIN. Therefore, when the term "PIN" is used today, it usually means high-grade PIN.

Prostatic Intraepithelial Neoplasia (PIN)

Prostatic intraepithelial neoplasia (PIN) is a kind of tissue that is not normal, but it is also not cancerous. (The term has replaced the words "dysplasia," "malignant transformation," and "intraductal carcinoma") Many doctors believe that PIN can go on to, or become associated with, prostate cancer.

Important things you need to know about PIN:

▶ The only way to detect it is by having a biopsy. (The same is true of prostate cancer.)

▶ It does not change the PSA level to any significant degree.

▶ It usually exists together with prostate cancer. Anywhere from 5% to 40% of the men with prostate cancer also have PIN.

▶ PIN increases with age and may be found up to five years before cancer of the prostate. The mean age of men with PIN is only 65, compared to a mean age of 70 for men with prostate cancer.

▶ PIN is more common in African-American men than in Caucasian men. It also seems to begin about 10 years earlier in African-Americans.

▶ If high-grade PIN is reported on the first biopsy, there is about a 50% chance that prostate cancer will be diagnosed on the next biopsy. The best thing to do if someone has been diagnosed with high-grade PIN is to have a repeat biopsy that includes tissue samples from both sides of the prostate, because cancer can occur away from the PIN area.

▶ There is a decrease in the number of cases and amount of PIN with hormonal therapy.

▶ Smoking

Numerous studies indicate either a slight prostate cancer risk or no risk at all for men who smoke cigarettes. Some recent studies suggest a possible increase in the risk of dying from prostate cancer if the man continues to smoke after diagnosis. One thing is known—smoking does not decrease the risk of getting prostate cancer, and it definitely increases the risk of lung cancer. So quitting smoking—or not starting—is a good idea.

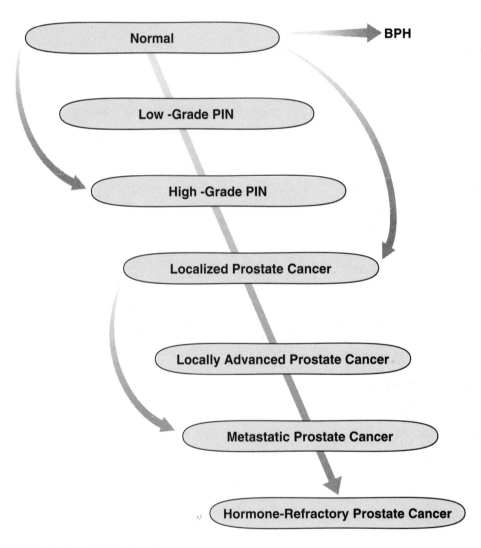

FIGURE C-1.—PIN chart.

Low-Grade PIN

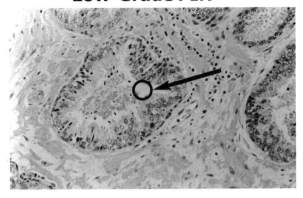

High-Grade PIN

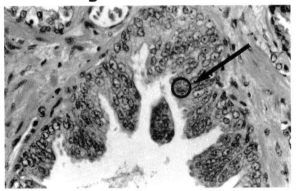

High-Grade PIN with Cancer

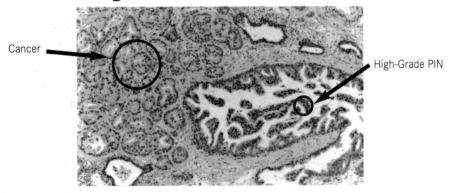

FIGURE C-2.—PIN slide views.

AAH Can Look Like Cancer

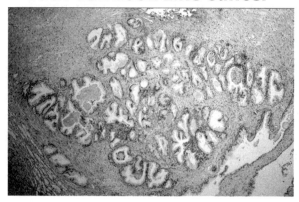

AAH with a Stain that Shows the Basal Layer

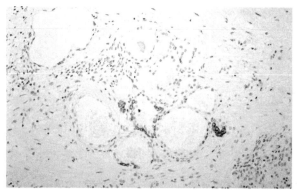

A Closer Look at the Basal Layer of AAH

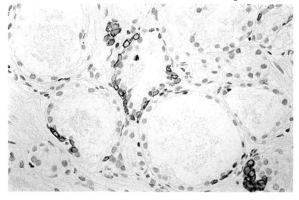

FIGURE C-3.—AAH slide views.

Atypical Adenomatous Hyperplasia (AAH)

Atypical adenomatous hyperplasia (AAH) are slightly abnormal cells that usually appear with benign prostatic hyperplasia (BPH) in an area of the prostate where few prostate cancers are found. AAH can look like cancer to a pathologist, but a test that looks for a "basal layer" can determine whether the cells are AAH or cancer. (The basal layer is disrupted or absent in cancer.) No one is sure whether having AAH puts someone at an increased risk for having prostate cancer.

► Vasectomy

A few years ago, the National Institutes of Health reviewed all the information concerning vasectomy and prostate cancer and found no relationship. Therefore, a vasectomy has not been determined to be a risk factor for prostate cancer, and it probably does not decrease the risk either.

► Hormone Levels

There is still a lot of work to be done in understanding the relationship between hormones and prostate cancer, but it is believed that high levels of testosterone are associated with an increased risk of prostate cancer, and low levels of testosterone are associated with a decreased risk of prostate cancer. The picture is more complex than that, however, and may involve other hormones and even enzymes that can change one hormone into another.

For example, men with higher levels of the hormone estradiol, a type of estrogen usually found in larger amounts in women, seem to be at a decreased risk for developing prostate cancer. Also, men with lower levels of sex hormone-binding globulin (SHBG), a protein in the bloodstream that binds to testosterone and other hormones, seem to be at an increased risk for prostate cancer. High levels of a hormone called insulin-like growth factor (IGF-1) may be a risk factor for prostate cancer but this needs to be further tested.

INFORMATION ABOUT NUTRITION, SUPPLEMENTS, AND PROSTATE CANCER

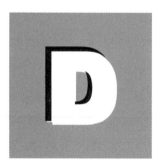

WHAT ARE THE SUPPLEMENTS TO TAKE TO EITHER PREVENT PROSTATE CANCER OR TO STOP IT FROM PROGRESSING?

FIRST THE ROLE OF SUPPLEMENTS MUST BE UNDERSTOOD, AND THEIR SAFE AND PROPER USE. UNLESS TAKEN CORRECTLY, THE BENEFITS OF SUPPLEMENTS CAN BE LOST AND THERE MAY BE SIDE EFFECTS.

> # Understand the Differences between
> # RDA, RDI, ODA, and ODI
>
> ## RDA—*Recommended Daily Allowance*
>
> The government established these allowances to represent dosages that may potentially eliminate the chances of contracting a rare nutritional disease. For example, 60 mg of vitamin C daily is the RDA to prevent diseases such as scurvy.
>
> ## RDI—*Recommended Daily Intake*
>
> These have been established by the government and in some cases have recently replaced the RDAs. Cross reference RDAs and RDIs, as they are not always the same.
>
> ## ODA—*Optimum Daily Allowance*
>
> This term is normally used to describe the maximum amount necessary to prevent a chronic disease. The ODA recommendations are usually much higher than the RDAs and RDIs.
>
> ## ODI—*Optimum Daily Intake*
>
> This term is interchangeable with ODA, it is simply a matter of preference.

▶ How Do Supplements Work to Fight or Prevent Cancer?

Generally, supplements and chemoprevention medicines (things that prevent cancer) fall into a class of chemicals called antioxidants. As the body metabolizes nutrients (breaks down food), bad molecules are formed inside the cell that damage the DNA as well as other parts of the cell. These bad molecules are often called free radicals. Chemoprevention medicines are antioxidants that fight free radicals from forming and damaging the body.

▶ Take Supplements with Caution

If someone followed the advice given by all the self-proclaimed "experts" or that found in supplement magazines, they could easily spend a lot of money. Supplements do not require FDA approval, so the FDA cannot regulate the manner in which they are advertised, other than to prevent manufacturers from making specific claims about a product. Anyone who is considering taking a supplement or changing their diet should make certain they are following the advice of someone who has objectively reviewed all of the studies on the supplement, vitamin, or diet.

There remains a tremendous amount of information yet to review regarding nutrition and supplements. For now, it is best to take advantage of what is known. For example, take the use of selenium as a treatment for prostate cancer. In clinical research trials, people who took 200 mcg per day of selenium did very well. Following this news, several supplement companies began manufacturing selenium at doses much higher than needed and with fancy additives such as zinc and a variety of herbs. This was done so that in marketing these supplements they could claim an overall healthful effect for the general population and therefore sell them to a larger market. However, these products have not been proven to be effective. Only those supplements proven effective in clinical studies should be taken. It may be a waste of money to purchase and consume unproven supplements with fancy additives.

▶ Take Supplements Correctly

Almost all supplements should be taken with a meal or up to 20 to 30 minutes before or after a meal. There are two simple reasons why. First, the body will absorb it better when it is taken with a meal. Vitamin E is a classic example: unless it is taken with food (or a small amount of fat), little to none of it is absorbed. Second, one of the most frequently cited reasons for not being able to tolerate a supplement is stomach upset. Selenium, taken on an empty stomach, can cause a lot of gas and stomach pain. This can be virtually eliminated in most cases if the supplement is taken at or close to mealtime.

It is generally good to divide the daily dosage. If, for example, the recommended dosage is 400 IU of vitamin E daily, 200 IU can be taken early in the day and 200 IU late in the day. Dividing the dosages allows the body to tolerate the supplement better and reduces any side effects. It will also allow the supplement to remain in the bloodstream for

24 hours, thereby providing the full benefit of the supplement. Either purchase smaller doses and take them twice per day or cut the pills in half.

It is a common misconception that if a supplement is good at recommended dosages, it is even better if consumed in large quantities. This is wrong as the body needs to adjust and tolerate supplements. Most medications are prescribed at a low dosage, and then if necessary the physician increases the dosage. It is no different with supplements. For example, if 800 IU of vitamin E is recommended to control hot flashes, begin with 200 IU, after a few weeks increase to 400 IU, after a few more weeks increase to 600 IU, and finally after a few more weeks increase to 800 IU. This gives the body time to adjust.

In general, people seem to believe that they can take a supplement for a few days and see an immediate result. This is rarely the case. Most supplements require a long-term commitment before any benefits are felt. Research clearly supports this.

Understand the Differences between IU, mg, and mcg

Dosages can be very confusing. Understand the dosage before purchasing and taking any supplement. IU stands for International Units and is usually applied to fat-soluble vitamins, such as A, D, E, and K. An IU is a measure of the potency of a supplement and is very different from milligrams or micrograms. For example, 50 mg of vitamin E is not necessarily equal to 50 IU of vitamin E. It is actually closer to 75 IU in some cases. The abbreviation "mg" stands for milligram, or one-thousandth of a gram. The abbreviation "mcg" stands for microgram and is equal to one-millionth of a gram. Take the time to understand the dosage levels.

IU	=	International Unit
mg	=	milligram (one-thousandth of a gram)
mcg	=	microgram (one-millionth of a gram)

▶ Get Good Advice about Nutrition and Supplements

Most doctors want to provide their patients with nutrition and supplement information, but they do not always know enough to thoroughly discuss these issues. For the most part it is because they were not provided these classes in medical school or residency. In general, physicians want to learn more about these subjects.

Store Supplements in a Cool, Dark, Dry Place

In order to make sure that supplements remain stable and do not expire early it is important to store them in the proper place. Never put them in the refrigerator—they will collect too much moisture. Do not place them on top of the refrigerator either, as it is too warm. Place them in a cupboard, in a medicine cabinet, or on top of the dining room or kitchen table, out of direct sunlight.

If someone lectures on a health-related topic and seems to push a product or supplement over and over again, ask if he or she has any financial interest or is involved with the company in any way. It's a good rule of thumb to research the speaker ahead of time. This is not meant to imply that if a financial interest in the product exists that the speaker is not to be trusted. However, for an objective perspective it is important to understand all the circumstances before making a commitment to a person or product.

In addition, if a health professional provides advice, is it realistic? Do they practice what they preach? Is the person mentally and physically healthy? Healthy behavior and

---

Supplements Should Only be Used when Natural Sources Are Difficult to Obtain

Fruits and vegetables are the best natural source of vitamins and minerals. Check the label and make sure the product is pure. Do not want to purchase anything with fillers, preservatives, or additives.

---

practices can be addictive and infectious. If the person does not serve as a healthy role model it will be more difficult to follow their advice.

Remember, it is impossible to copy one aspect of healthy behavior from another culture and experience the same results. For example, simply drinking green tea because the Japanese do is not going to produce the same results. The consumption of green tea is only one aspect of their culture. The same study says that the more green tea that is consumed, the less likely someone is to smoke and the more likely to exercise, eat, and drink soy products, and maintain a healthy weight. A healthy culture carries with it an almost infinite number of healthy behaviors, some measurable and some not measurable. It is important for someone to look at their overall lifestyle, including profession, relationships, and hobbies, etc., as having an impact on their general health.

SUPPLEMENTS USED FOR PROSTATE CANCER PREVENTION AND TREATMENT

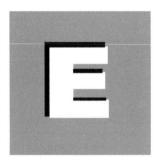

IT IS IMPORTANT TO NOTE THAT **NO** DIET OR SUPPLEMENT OR CHEMOPREVENTION AGENT HAS EVER BEEN PROVEN TO PREVENT PROSTATE CANCER. THE FOLLOWING IS A DISCUSSION OF THE SUPPLEMENTS, NUTRIENTS, AND HOLISTIC APPROACHES USED FOR PROSTATE CANCER AND WHETHER OR NOT THEY MAY BE USEFUL IN PROSTATE CANCER PREVENTION AND TREATMENT.

General Recommendations

One of the most effective ways of dealing with prostate cancer treatment is to remember the following:

▶ Be mentally prepared and healthy about treatment. Determine what will help accomplish this goal and do it. It may enhance the chances of a positive result.

▶ Do not be discouraged about reducing supplements during procedures. Nutritional levels can be maintained through healthy eating.

▶ The National Cancer Institute advocates at least five servings of fruits and vegetables per day. One way to accomplish this is to drink smoothies. Smoothies can provide daily servings of fruit, as well as anticancer compounds, vitamins, minerals, and fiber. The flaxseed and soy protein powder in each smoothie will provide plant estrogens and fiber.

▶ One week before and two weeks after a procedure, eat in the healthiest way possible. Try to follow the guidelines below:

> Heart healthy = Prostate healthy
> Low saturated fat intake—minimal meat
> Exercise
> Increase consumption of fruits and vegetables
> Fish—several times a week
> Drink plenty of fruit and vegetable juices
> Alcohol—limited or not at all
> Make certain your diet contains soy and flaxseed
> Drink several cups of green tea daily
> Avoid fast food meals—they provide little nutritional Value

▶ Talk to the doctor about taking a general multivitamin (with B-vitamins, 400 IU of vitamin D, and 400 IU of folic acid). It might also be a very good idea to talk to a nutritionist.

▶ Sleep at least 6 to 8 hours a night.

▶ Keep stress to a minimum.

▶ Socialize, and discuss treatment.

▶ Beta-Carotene, Vitamin A, and Retinoids

Beta-Carotene

Carotenoids are antioxidants that play an important role in helping prevent various diseases, including some cancers. They are one of a group of pigments (organic coloring matter in the body), ranging in color from light yellow to red. The most commonly recognized is beta-carotene, which is found in carrots, but other carotenoids include lycopene (found in tomatoes) and lutein (found in spinach). Carotenoids are commonly found in foods such as carrots, tomatoes, and spinach. The greater the intensity of color in the fruit or vegetable, the higher the amount of beta-carotene it contains.

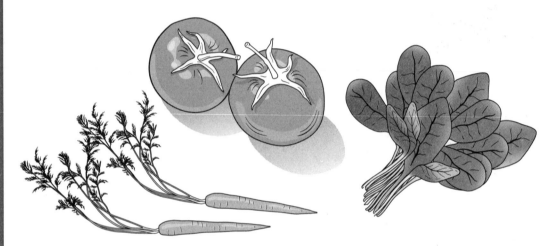

FIGURE E-1.— Tomatoes, carrots, and spinach.

Vitamin A

Vitamin A is formed in the body from carotenoid precursors. It is essential for normal growth and development, the normal function and integrity of epithelial tissue (cells that form the outer surface of the body and line the body cavities and principle tubes and passageways leading to the exterior), and normal tooth and bone development.

Retinoids

Retinoids are a class of compounds that include vitamin A. One retinoid, 4-hydroxyphenyl retinamide (4-HPR) is derived from vitamin A and has been successful in preventing some prostate tumors in animals. They are currently associated with quite a few side effects—such as headaches, skin, liver, and vision problems—but may develop as a viable option within a short period of time if the side effects can be reduced.

The supplement form of beta-carotene and/or vitamin A accomplishes little. However, foods rich in vitamin A provide a number of antioxidants and other potential anticancer compounds. Fruits and vegetables eaten on a daily basis will provide plenty of beta-carotene and vitamin A.

The general conclusion from all of the studies on beta-carotene is that there is a chance of reducing prostate cancer if a diet that is low in fat and high in vitamin-rich fruits and vegetables is followed, but no specific recommendations are available at this time.

The Differences between Fat-Soluble and Water-Soluble Vitamins

There are primarily four fat-soluble vitamins:

Vitamin A
Vitamin D
Vitamin E
Vitamin K

Fat-soluble vitamins are stored in fatty tissue. The body normally stores them in large quantities.

Most of the remaining vitamins are water-soluble. Water-soluble vitamins are not stored in large quantities. When the body takes in more water-soluble vitamins than it needs, the excess is eliminated as waste. As far as research has shown, the only noticeable difference between fat-soluble and water-soluble vitamins is that fat-soluble vitamins require a little dietary fat to be adequately absorbed.

▶ B-Vitamins

B-vitamins are a group of water-soluble vitamins isolated from liver, yeast, and other sources. They are important in carbohydrate metabolism and in the normal functioning of nervous tissue. B-vitamins are popular because they provide energy and are needed for the proper metabolism of sugars (carbohydrates), fats, and proteins. During periods of stress the body loses vitamin B, thus it is important to obtain vitamin B during stressful periods. Vitamin B also helps to reduce high levels of homocysteine (an amino acid), which may increase the risk of a heart attack, and may be involved in reducing a number of cancers.

Over the past few years, four of the B-vitamins have received a lot of attention as a result of their ability to reduce heart disease and, potentially, cancer. The fabulous four are B_3, B_6, B_{12}, and folic acid. Each is easily obtained through dietary food sources. Vegetables, fruits, and beans are good sources of niacin, folic acid, B_6, and B_{12}. They may be taken in a general multivitamin or a multiple B-vitamin.

Unfortunately, there have been very few studies on the effect of B-vitamins and prostate cancer. Therefore, no conclusions about their usefulness in preventing prostate cancer can be drawn at this time.

▶ Coenzyme Q (CoQ$_{10}$, CoQ, Coenzyme Q$_{10}$, Ubiquinone)

Coenzyme Q (CoQ$_{10}$, CoQ, Coenzyme Q$_{10}$, Ubiquinone) is integral to energy production by various cells of the body, especially the heart cells. It has received much attention recently because it also seems to function as a strong antioxidant.

The human body is normally very adept at manufacturing Coenzyme Q. The combination of tyrosine (an amino acid found in many foods), vitamins B_2, B_6, B_{12}, niacinamide, pantothenic acid, folic acid, and vitamin C is used by the body in the creation of Coenzyme Q.

Several laboratory studies have shown that Coenzyme Q may be helpful for cancer patients who are undergoing chemotherapy. In fact, these studies suggest that it be taken while undergoing any type of chemotherapeutic treatment that might also be toxic to the heart. Keep in mind that there is very limited data currently available. Please talk to a doctor if you wish to take Coenzyme Q for the side effects caused by a chemotherapeutic drug. A number of other studies have indicated that Coenzyme Q is not effective. One randomized placebo-controlled clinical trial showed that men who received 90 mg of Coenzyme Q a day did not experience a protective effect from oxidative DNA damage when compared to the control group. In fact, the control group (those taking the placebo) had a better result. There does not appear to be a role for Coenzyme Q in preventing prostate cancer at this time.

Coenzyme Q, much like vitamin K, can interfere with prescribed blood thinners, and cholesterol-reducing drugs can lower blood Coenzyme Q levels. Anyone who is taking a prescription anticoagulant (Warfarin), should not take supplemental Coenzyme Q or the effectiveness of the anticoagulant will be reduced.

► DHEA

Dehydroepiandosterone (DHEA) is a hormone manufactured by humans. Hormones are compounds normally secreted in the blood in very tiny amounts. These hormones travel to other parts of the body to cause an action or actions. For example, the hormone testosterone, largely manufactured in the testicles, travels throughout the body and causes multiple effects, ranging from a deeper voice, to hair growth or loss, to determining the sex of a baby. Hormones like testosterone have local effects (e.g., assistance with proper sperm function) and distant effects (e.g., influencing the release of other hormones in the brain).

DHEAS is the same compound as DHEA with a sulfate (S) attached. Both DHEA and DHEAS are manufactured in the adrenal glands, located on top of the kidneys. Smaller amounts are manufactured by the brain, gonads, and skin. The DHEA present in the liver and kidneys also creates DHEAS. DHEAS is by far the most abundant hormone in the human body. Both DHEA and DHEAS are considered weak androgens and they are not as powerful as testosterone.

While many claims have been made, no benefits for DHEA/DHEAS have been proven in significant randomized, placebo-controlled clinical trials. The FDA has not approved the use of this hormone by physicians for any condition, and in fact banned the sale of DHEA in 1985. The ban was lifted in 1994 with the passage of the Dietary Supplement Health and Education Act. (The Dietary Supplement Health and Education Act places the burden on the FDA to prove that a nutritional supplement is harmful.)

DHEA/DHEAS should not be used for the following reasons:

- ► DHEA/DHEAS are converted to testosterone.
- ► It has increased tumor growth in clinical trials.
- ► The limited amount of data available regarding DHEA/DHEAS and prostate cancer makes it safer to emphasize the drawbacks rather than positives until more studies are complete.

Types of Fat

Fat is a group of compounds composed of one or more fatty acids and glycerol, a compound present in fat. When fats from food are digested, they are broken down into different components. The body changes these components so that they can be carried through the blood.

Fatty Acids, the building blocks of fat, are composed of chains of carbon, hydrogen, and oxygen. They differ from one another in two ways: the length of the chain and whether they are saturated or not. Most fats are a mixture of the three major types of fatty acids: saturated, monounsaturated, and polyunsaturated.

Triglycerides, composed of three fatty acids, are a major component of the storage of fat in the body. Most dietary fat is in the form of triglycerides. Individuals with a higher level of triglycerides are at an increased risk for heart disease.

Saturated Fat contains the maximum number of hydrogen molecules on its chain. Saturated fats, if eaten over a long period of time, can increase the risk of heart disease. Common sources of saturated fats: animal fat, especially from beef; cheeses made from whole milk or cream; butter; palm oil; and coconut oil.

Hydrogenation is the process of adding hydrogen to an unsaturated fat to create a solid **saturated fat**. Hydrogenated fat is another name for a saturated fat product on a food label.

Monounsaturated Fat or fatty acid molecules have one pair of hydrogen atoms on the chain that is missing. Monounsaturated fat is not as compact as saturated fat and is considered a little healthier. Common sources of monounsaturated fat: nuts, pork, oatmeal, canola oil, olive oil, and peanut oil.

In a **Polyunsaturated Fat** at least two pairs of hydrogen atoms are missing from the chain. Polyunsaturated fats may reduce blood lipids, but an excess may also lower the protective cholesterol (HDL) as well. There are also a number of specialized polyunsaturated fatty acids, such as omega-3, omega-6, and trans fatty acids. Common sources of polyunsaturated fat: soybeans, squash, sweet potatoes, fish, and most vegetable oils.

Omega-3 Fatty Acids are a special type of polyunsaturated fat. For example, linolenic acid (an essential fatty acid available only through diet), is a common omega-3 fatty acid. Other sources include cold-water fish, seafood, and fish oil supplements. Flaxseed and flaxseed oil are the largest sources of omega-3 fatty acids.

Trans Fatty Acids are another type of polyunsaturated fat. They do not occur naturally in plants and only a small amount is found in animals. Trans fatty acids are processed, and have been hydrogenated to make the fat or vegetable oil more solid. Margarine is a good example. Studies have shown that these fats can raise cholesterol levels in the blood.

Most oils contain a mixture of fatty acids. Fatty acids, regardless of where they come from, are the building blocks of fat. Often people think that certain oils are very healthy, such as olive oil. One tablespoon of olive oil contains approximately 14 grams of total fat (mostly monounsaturated), two of which are saturated fat grams.

▶ Fat

Fatty tissue or adipose tissue are medical terms for body fat. Energy is normally stored in body fat. It also serves as protection for several organs and can insulate the body from different temperatures. However, an excessive amount of body fat is harmful. It has been linked to various diseases, such as heart disease, cancer, high blood pressure, and type II diabetes.

Dietary fat is the fat found in various foods. Fat from the diet helps provide energy and essential fatty acids. (Some fatty acids cannot be made in the body. They can only be obtained from the diet, and are essential especially for children.) It also carries vitamins A, D, E, and K.

It makes a huge difference whether the fat is saturated, monounsaturated, or polyunsaturated. Eskimos eat as much, if not more fat than the average American, but the kind of fat they consume is different. Most of their fat intake is from fish. The omega-3 fatty acids in the fish may provide benefits beyond what is currently known. Researchers have determined that saturated fat intake may increase the risk of cancer (breast, colon, and prostate). Laboratory studies examining diets and prostate cancer risk in humans have shown an increased risk of prostate cancer with a high fat intake.

Fat should not be eliminated from a diet completely. Fat is absolutely necessary for energy and for other vital functions. A generally agreed upon healthy amount of dietary fat is 20% of daily intake, with as little as possible from saturated fat—less than 10% of total daily fat intake.

Low-fat foods may also contain other potentially protective components. For example, fruits and vegetables contain numerous antioxidants, fiber, and other compounds that can potentially inhibit the growth of prostate tumors.

▶ Fiber

Several studies have shown that dietary fiber can lower the risk of prostate cancer and/or prostate cancer progression. Data on dietary fiber found in fruits and vegetables indicates that this is the better route for good health. In a study with vegetarians who consumed fiber from natural sources it was discovered they had lower levels of testosterone than nonvegetarians. This seems to indicate that dietary fiber may work by lowering levels of certain hormones (e.g., testosterone) that promote prostate cancer growth and progression. A diet that includes natural fiber increases the chance of good health and may reduce the risk of prostate cancer.

▶ Flaxseed

Phytoestrogen is a term for foods or plants that contain a natural source of estrogen. Flaxseed is an excellent source of phytoestrogen. Flaxseed is a tiny seed that is used to make linseed oil and is the largest source of "lignans," another class of phytoestrogens. Lignans are also found in a variety of other foods, such as lentils and garlic.

Flaxseed is available in a variety of forms: plain flaxseed, flaxseed meal, flaxseed flour (or powder), flaxseed capsules, and flaxseed oil. Books, magazines, and health professionals are touting flaxseed oil and capsules as a sort of cure-all, for everything from

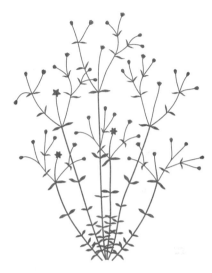

FIGURE E-2.— Flaxseed

allergies to cancer. Use extreme caution with both the oil and the capsules, as they contain a high amount of fat.

Flaxseed has undergone very few studies when it comes to disease, especially cancer. However, the early data indicates that it may be beneficial against cancer. The preliminary studies indicate that flaxseeds may possibly bring some benefit by:

▶ High in fiber (decreases cholesterol levels)
▶ Acting as estrogenic agents in some cases.
▶ Acting as antiestrogenic agents in other cases.
▶ Acting as strong antioxidants.
▶ Blocking tumor growth.
▶ Blocking the conversion of hormones to other hormones that may stimulate cancer growth.
▶ Inhibiting angiogenesis (or the growth of new blood vessels by tumors).
▶ Increasing the amount of sex hormone-binding globulin (also known as SHBG). SHBG can bind to hormones and make them less available to other parts of the body and cancers (therefore, the less the amount of hormone(s) available to the cancer, the less fuel it has to grow).
▶ Acting as immune system enhancers.
▶ Being a good source of omega-3 fatty acids, mostly alpha-linolenic acid, which has been found in numerous studies to possibly reduce the risk of cancer.

▶ Garlic

Garlic is one of more than 500 members of the allium plant family. Several other well-known members of the family include: chives, onions, shallots, and leeks. A recent study discovered an association between increased consumption of both natural garlic and garlic supplements and a lower risk of prostate cancer. The study found that individuals who consumed natural garlic at least twice a week had a lower risk of prostate cancer. It also determined that individuals who took garlic supplements along with natural garlic also had

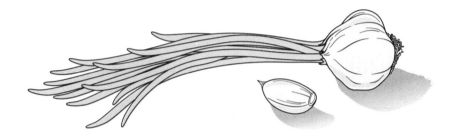

FIGURE E-3.—Garlic

a lower risk, although not as low as the garlic only group. In conclusion, this study found that men who consumed natural garlic, vitamin B-6, beans, or peas on a regular basis had a lower risk of prostate cancer. No specific recommendations, however, can be made at this time.

▶ Lycopene

Lycopene is one of the hundreds of carotenoids found in nature. Carotenoids are natural pigments thought to be helpful in the prevention of some diseases, including cancer. It is the carotenoids in tomatoes that make them red. Most carotenoids, including lycopene, are not converted into vitamin A. Laboratory studies have proven lycopene to be one of the strongest antioxidants in nature. It is found in very high concentration in tomatoes, tomato products, and several other foods. In fact, more than 80% of the lycopene intake in the United States comes from tomato products. Cooked tomatoes contain even more lycopene. The heat releases lycopene from the food's specific storage area and makes it more available to be absorbed by the body.

In a study of 14,000 men who ate tomatoes more than five times a week (versus those who ate less than one serving a week), prostate cancer risk was reduced. The largest tomato and prostate cancer study showed a 35% decrease in prostate cancer risk among individuals who ate more than ten servings a week of tomato products. It was further determined from this study that the consumption of tomato products also decreased the risk of being diagnosed with advanced or aggressive prostate cancer. Tomato sauce was associated with the lowest prostate cancer risk, with tomatoes and pizza showing a moderate decrease while tomato juice provided little protection. While no clear recommendations can be made at this time, lycopene may play a role in preventing prostate cancer. There is currently very little information available on lycopene supplements.

▶ Melatonin

Melatonin, a hormone, is manufactured in the pineal gland, which is in the center of the brain. Melatonin is key in functions such as puberty, reproduction, sleep cycles, moods, cancer growth, and aging. The formation of melatonin is stimulated by darkness and inhibited by ordinary light.

Researchers have found that Melatonin can:

▶ Decrease levels of luteinizing hormone (LH) in the brain. LH stimulates the production of testosterone in the testicles.

▶ Serve as a strong antioxidant. One study found melatonin to be more effective than other antioxidants, such as vitamin E, in protecting DNA and other components of the body from oxidative damage. (These antioxidant properties are normally found when melatonin levels are high as a result of melatonin supplements and not from the levels generated by the pineal gland.)

▶ Potentially boost the immune system. In fact, certain cells in the immune system have receptors for melatonin in order to enhance their function. A number of animal studies have shown that melatonin may also be involved in enhancing other areas of the immune system.

Several clinical studies have shown that individuals who take even small amounts of supplemental melatonin (5 mg) are able to increase both sleep and dream time. Other studies have shown that much lower levels (0.1 to 1 mg) may do the same. In fact, 1 to 2 mg, taken for at least 3 to 4 weeks seems to increase the quantity and quality of sleep for insomniacs. Another clinical study observed international flight crew members who took 5 mg of melatonin at bedtime on the day of their return home and for five days afterwards. Researchers found that jet lag, sleep problems, and daytime fatigue decreased among those who took the melatonin and not the placebo. Optimum dosage and use are still being carefully studied.

Very small and preliminary studies have suggested that taking melatonin may increase the effectiveness of hormone therapy for advanced prostate cancer patients. No recommendations can be given at this time.

▶ PC-SPES and PC-SPES-like Products (PC-Calm, . . .)

PC-SPES (the PC stands for "prostate cancer," and spes is the Latin word for "hope") is a combination of eight herbs that are used in Chinese medicine to treat cancer. Each 320-mg capsule contains a combination of the following herbs:

> *Isatis indigotica* (da qing ye)
> *Glycyrrhiza glabra* and *Glycyrrhiza uralensis* (gan cao)—licorice
> *Panax pseudo-Ginseng* (san qi)—ginseng
> *Ganoderma lucidum* (ling zhi)
> *Scutellaria baicalensis* (huang qin)—skull cap
> *Dendranthema morifolium Tzvel*—chrysanthemum
> *Rabdosia rebescens*
> *Serenoa repens*—saw palmetto

PC-SPES has been advertised as a nonestrogenic food supplement (it contains no estrogen), but several of its components appear to have definite estrogenic activity. Intake of PC-SPES substantially decreases testosterone and PSA levels and has side effects such as breast enlargement, breast tenderness, loss of libido, and blood clots.

Recently, the California Department of Health may have found the blood thinner Warfarin as well as other medicines in PC-SPES. This potentially is a troublesome finding and it remains to be seen what role PC-SPES has as a preventive or treatment agent against prostate cancer. At this time, PC-SPES has been taken off the market. Other estrogenic supplements (e.g., PC-Calm) are being marketed in its place. PC-Calm contains 6 of the herbs found in PC-SPES plus 4 additional ones. The identity of the herbs in PC-Calm is not clear.

▶ Resveratrol

Resveratrol, a polyphenol, is commonly found in grapes and wine, especially red wine. Laboratory studies have shown that it may help decrease PSA secretion and inhibit the growth of hormone-sensitive and hormone-insensitive prostate cancer cells. Again, more research needs to be conducted with both animals and humans before specific recommendations can be made. However, there have been a number of studies that have shown that moderate wine or alcohol consumption may protect against heart disease, by increasing HDL levels (the good cholesterol), for example. There has never been a strong connection made between alcohol consumption and prostate cancer risk or progression. Even among men who were found to consume 57 or more drinks a week (a drink being equal to a glass of wine, beer, or shot of whiskey) for more than 10 years, there was no additional risk. The only slight risk was for men who consumed 120 drinks a week.

▶ Selenium

Selenium is a trace mineral. Selenium is a popular antioxidant because it works directly with an enzyme in the body to prevent free radical damage.

The first double-blind, placebo-controlled cancer prevention study to test the effectiveness of selenium was conducted at the University of Arizona.

There was:

- ▶ A 37% decrease in overall cancer incidences.
- ▶ A 46% decrease in lung cancer.
- ▶ A 58% decrease in colorectal cancer.
- ▶ A 63% decrease in prostate cancer.

It is possible that selenium and vitamin E may work better together to enhance each other's effect at reducing the risk of prostate cancer. Low levels of selenium have been associated with a higher risk of some cancers, including prostate cancer. A dose of 200 mcg a day of selenium has been associated with a reduction in the number of localized and advanced prostate cancers. Dietary intake of selenium-rich foods is linked to a 50% to 75% decrease in advanced prostate cancers.

A dose of 200 mcg of selenium daily is inexpensive and safe. Selenium is difficult to obtain from foods in large quantities.

▶ Shark Cartilage

The skeleton of a shark is composed of cartilage, not bone. The shark cartilage supplement is made by drying the cartilage, pulverizing it into a powder, and then packaging it in capsule form. The theory behind shark cartilage supplements is that they have shown limited potential as an antiangiogenic agent. Cancerous tumors require blood vessels and nutrients to grow. An antiangiogenic agent restricts blood vessel growth and therefore the supply of nutrients to a tumor. In the few studies that have been completed to test this theory, the shark cartilage itself has been used, not the supplement. Shark cartilage may also contain antiinflammatory properties and the ability to reduce damage caused by free radicals. Overall research is very limited, but at this time there is no reason to believe that shark cartilage prevents or treats prostate cancer.

▶ Soy

Soy contains phytoestrogens. The soybean is the source of many different soy products. It is important to read the label of a "soy" product. Many of them, for example soy sauce, actually contain very little soy.

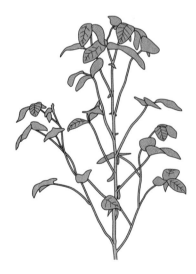

FIGURE E-4.—Soybean

Isoflavones are the most common type of phytoestrogen. The two major isoflavones in soy are genistein and daidzein. Isoflavones are found in many different plants, including fruits and vegetables, especially leguminous plants, which contain a large concentration of soy. Soybeans (or roasted soybeans) are usually the largest source of plant estrogen, while soy protein powder and tempeh contain a moderate amount, and soy milk contains a small amount. The more the soybean is manipulated, the more likely it is that plant estrogen is lost.

The prostate cancer death rate in Asian countries is very low compared to that of the United States. For example, prostate cancer death rates are somewhere between four to seven times lower in Japan than in the United States. Studies have shown that men in Asian countries consume on the average of about 50 to 100 mg of isoflavones (soy) daily compared to approximately 1 to 5 mg per day for American men.

Laboratory studies have shown that plant estrogens may also prevent prostate cancer by:

▶ Decreasing blood androgen (male hormone) levels.

▶ Increasing the concentration of sex hormone-binding globulin (SHBG), a protein that can bind to male hormones and prevent them from being used by the prostate to stimulate the growth of cancer.

▶ Binding to hormone receptors, so that even if a hormone is available it cannot bind to the prostate.

▶ Inhibiting 5-alpha-reductase, an enzyme in the prostate that converts natural testosterone into a more powerful testosterone called dihydrotestosterone (DHT).

▶ Restricting other enzymes associated with cell growth.

▶ Causing direct tumor destruction such as antiangiogenesis, which does not allow the cancer to make more blood vessels (thus starving the tumor).

▶ Decreasing IGF-1—increased levels of IGF-1 have recently been shown to be a potential marker for increased risk of prostate cancer in several human clinical studies.

Asian men also have a low fat intake as compared to men in the United States and drink much more green tea. However, it appears that a diet high in soy may protect against prostate cancer.

▶ Tea

Green, Oolong, and Black Teas

The tea plant, which can grow to an average height of 30 feet, is the source for all three types of tea: green, oolong, and black. The only difference between the three types is how they are processed. Green tea leaves are lightly steamed or dried—unfermented. Oolong tea is partially fermented. Black tea is completely fermented.

During the oxidation process enzymes in the tea change the polyphenols (the compounds in tea that make it healthy) into less active components. In green tea the process of steaming the leaves prevents oxidation from occurring. These polyphenols also provide many antioxidant and anticancer properties.

Flavonoids are the most abundant polyphenol in green tea. A flavonoid is one of a group of compounds found in plants. There are more than 4,000 known flavonoids. They are responsible for the deep colors of berries and are found in some fruits, vegetables, nuts, seeds, grains, legumes, coffee, wine, and of course, tea. Flavanols, also known as catechins, are a type of flavonoid that has received a great deal of attention for its anticancer effects. Green tea contains about 30% to 40% catechins, while black tea contains only 5% to 10% after the fermentation process. Oolong tea falls in between green and black tea in terms of the compounds it contains. Catechins have been shown to kill cancer cells in the laboratory and can inhibit the enzyme 5-alpha-reductase, which converts testosterone into DHT (a more potent form of testosterone). Populations with lower levels of 5-alpha-reductase seem to have lower rates of prostate cancer. In fact, the largest clinical

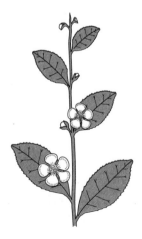

FIGURE E-5.—Tea plant

study (The Prostate Cancer Prevention Trial) is currently being conducted to determine whether a drug can lower the risk of prostate cancer by inhibiting this enzyme.

Essiac Tea

The four primary herbs found in Essiac tea are: burdock root (*Arctium lappa*); Indian rhubarb (*Rheum palmatum*); sheep sorrel (*Rumex acetosella*); and inner bark of the slippery elm (*Ulmus fulva* or *Ulmus rubra*). Four secondary ingredients found in similar products are: blessed thistle, kelp, red clover, and watercress. Advocates claim that if Essiac tea is taken during cancer treatments (i.e., chemotherapy or radiation therapy) the tea boosts the immune system, increases appetite, and helps reduce pain. There are also claims that it may decrease the size of various tumors and keep people alive longer. Most of the individuals using these teas today are doing so with conventional treatments and as supportive care for terminal disease.

Kombucha Tea

The kombucha mushroom, also called the Manchurian or kargasok mushroom, has been used in China and Russia for thousands of years. The kombucha is commonly referred to as a mushroom, but it is actually a combination of lichen, bacteria, and yeast. The kombucha is not eaten, but rather made into tea through a fermentation process. The daughter mushrooms, produced during the process, can be used to make more tea. This tea is believed to contain a number of nutrients and other healthy ingredients that may be useful in combating various diseases and may also provide a natural energy boost. Keep in mind that these are only claims and that they have not been scientifically researched. Since this tea is made in a unique way, it may be difficult to find.

► Vitamin C

Vitamin C is a water-soluble vitamin and easily absorbed. Vitamin C is not stored in large amounts in the body, although this does not mean that excess quantities are harmless. Vitamin C is sometimes referred to as ascorbic acid. Low intake of vitamin C has been related to a higher risk of nonhormone-dependent cancers. For example, cancers of the esophagus, oral cavity, and stomach, have been related to lower intakes of vitamin C. The generally accepted theory is that fruits and vegetables that contain high levels of vitamin C act together to provide anticancer benefits. However, there is no data that vitamin C is beneficial in preventing prostate cancer.

▶ Vitamin D and Calcium

Vitamin D has many functions, one of which is to signal the intestines to absorb calcium. It is important that both vitamin D and calcium are obtained. They need each other in order to produce the maximum effect in the body.

Osteoporosis is a weakness in the bones, or actual bone loss. As men and women age they are at an increased risk for this disease, especially women. Most bone loss with osteoporosis occurs in areas of the body that absorb stress or weight, such as the hips, ribs, and spinal area. There are many possible reasons for an increased risk of osteoporosis. One is low intake of calcium.

Two things happen simultaneously when a man ages. First, there is an increased risk of being diagnosed with prostate cancer, and second, the ability to manufacture vitamin D from sun exposure diminishes. Race also plays a part in the risk of prostate cancer. African-American men have an increased risk of being diagnosed with prostate cancer. This may be due in part to the fact that there is more melanin in African-American skin than, for example, Caucasian skin. Melanin blocks the body's ability to create vitamin D. Asian men obtain more vitamin D from fish than American men and have a lower risk of prostate cancer. Fresh tuna—a favorite of the Japanese—provides more than 16,000 IU of vitamin D per gram of fish. Individuals living in the northern areas of the United States have more trouble making vitamin D from exposure to the sun. To further complicate the situation, the winter sun in these northern areas is not intense enough to cause the body to manufacture adequate levels of vitamin D.

Studies have found that increased amounts of calcium intake may also be associated with a higher risk of prostate cancer. The body is sensitive to very high and very low levels of vitamins and minerals and tries to adjust each to a normal level. High intake of calcium may cause vitamin D levels to decrease. This is called a "feedback mechanism." If, for example, the body has too much calcium, it responds by lowering the level of vitamin D in order not to absorb the excess calcium. This is a signal (feedback) to the body to reduce the level of vitamin D.

The problem with too much vitamin D is that it can cause hypercalcemia (too much calcium in the blood). This is a dangerous condition. Excess calcium may be deposited in blood vessels and organs, thereby creating blockage in these areas.

Taking a daily multivitamin that contains approximately 400 IU of vitamin D is a good idea. Walk in the sun for at least 10 to 15 minutes three times a week. Eat one or two servings of fish (stay away from fish oil supplements) weekly unless otherwise instructed by the doctor. Consider increasing supplemental vitamin D intake to 800 IU during the fall and winter. Use skim or soy milk and products that are fortified with vitamin D. The doctor should be informed if someone is taking supplemental vitamin D.

► Vitamin E

Vitamin E is a general name for a group of compounds classified as either tocopherols or tocotrienols. Natural sources of vitamin E tend to increase fat intake. The best source of vitamin E is a supplement. Supplemental vitamin E comes from either natural or synthetic sources.

A Finnish clinical trial recently changed the perception of vitamin E's role in prostate cancer. In the trial, 29,133 Finnish male smokers, aged 50 to 69, were randomly assigned to receive either synthetic vitamin E (50 IU), beta-carotene (20 mg), both, or a placebo every day for 5 to 8 years. The men in the vitamin E group had a 32% lower risk of prostate cancer and a 41% lower risk of dying from prostate cancer within two years of the beginning of the trial.

The confusion over vitamin E seems to be regarding proper dosage. It is generally accepted that 800 IU is safe for older adults without disease. No adverse effects on body weight or lipid and blood cell profiles are experienced at this dosage. However, if 50 IU of vitamin E (synthetic) was found to be effective (in the Finnish trial) in adequately reducing prostate cancer incidences and deaths, why increase the dosage? Until more studies are complete it is advisable to remain with the lower dosage, unless the doctor recommends a high dosage to treat a specific condition, such as hot flashes.

► Zinc

Zinc, a mineral, is responsible for many functions in the human body. It is present in all organs, tissues, and fluids. Nearly 90% of the body's zinc is located in the bones and muscles. The normal prostate contains a large amount of zinc and prostate cancer cells do not. Zinc is necessary for the proper function of many enzymes and hormones in the body. Normally about 0.5 mg of zinc is lost from the body every day, but this is easily replaced by dietary sources. Zinc is also found in all types of fish, shellfish, beans, nuts, seeds, whole grains, and meats. There is no evidence that a person needs to take supplemental zinc.

▶ Aspirin (NSAIDs) and Prescription COX-2 Inhibitors (Celebrex, Vioxx, . . .)

If your doctor believes you qualify for aspirin (NSAIDs) therapy, ask him or her about newer evidence that may suggest that it reduces the risk of prostate cancer. Keep in mind that these products may have serious long term side effects (ulcers and/or internal bleeding), therefore, you should not begin taking these products without talking with your doctor first. Similar rules generally apply with the use of COX-2 inhibitors except they may have a lower rate of gastrointestinal side effects but these drugs are expensive, do not cause blood thinning, and may not have any impact on your risk of cardiovascular disease. Again, talk with your doctor about the advantages and disadvantages of these over the counter products and prescription medications.

Section

2

Finding

Prostate

Cancer

THE PROSTATE GLAND AND ITS FUNCTIONS

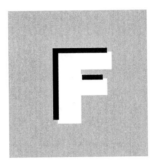

Cancer that is confined to the prostate displays few, if any, symptoms. There are some symptoms of general, noncancerous prostate problems that sometimes also appear with prostate cancer—usually some form of difficulty with the bladder and urinating. But it's important to remember that the presence of these symptoms does not mean someone has cancer. In fact, such symptoms are more common to an enlarged prostate, [benign prostate hyperplasia or benign prostatic hypertrophy (BPH)] or to inflammation of the prostate (prostatitis, which is usually caused by an infection). Basically, there are no urinary symptoms that can be used to definitively diagnose cancer of the prostate. The only way to truly diagnose prostate cancer is through a biopsy.

If prostate cancer advances to the seminal vesicles, it can lead to blood in the seminal fluid and/or a decrease in the amount of seminal fluid that is released after ejaculation. If the cancer advances to the nerve bundles around the prostate, impotence may be experienced. And if cancer has spread to the bones, there may be bone or back pain and fatigue. However, these symptoms are not specific to prostate cancer.

So, if someone has prostate cancer, it is likely that the individual will not have symptoms, and if there are symptoms, such as difficulties with urination, they may well be caused by other conditions. The rule is to have regular prostate checkups and have any urinary difficulty treated by a physician. The physician will probably perform a digital rectal exam (DRE), conduct a prostate-specific antigen (PSA) test, or, in some situations, perform a transrectal ultrasound (TRUS) to find the source of the problem.

▶ What is the Anatomy of the Prostate?

The following information will help someone understand a visit to the doctor. Open discussions with the doctor are a critical part of treatment. The information will help make those discussions clear and productive.

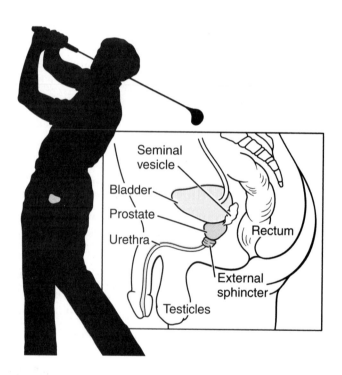

FIGURE F-1.—Anatomy of the Prostate Gland.

▶ The Zones of the Prostate

Only men have a prostate gland. Its purpose is to secrete about one-third of the fluid that carries sperm during ejaculation, or orgasm. The rest of the fluid is secreted by the two seminal vesicles, which lie on opposite sides of the prostate. Sperm itself is produced by the testicles, which also make the male hormone testosterone.

The prostate sits deep within the body, just below the bladder and above the rectum. The adult prostate is made up of three major zones: peripheral, central, and transition.

The Peripheral Zone

The largest of the three, the peripheral zone (PZ) makes up about two-thirds of the prostate. It encompasses the back and sides of the gland, from the bottom (also called the "apex") almost all the way to the top (also called the "base"). This may sound upside down, but the bottom of the prostate has more of a pointed end, hence the name "apex," while the top is wide and flat and sits below the bladder—hence the name "base."

When a physician inserts an index finger into the rectum to conduct a digital rectal exam (DRE), only the PZ can be felt. This is where the majority of prostate cancers begin. However, prostate cancers can also begin in the other two zones, which cannot be reached with a DRE. In order to examine those areas, an ultrasound machine must be used.

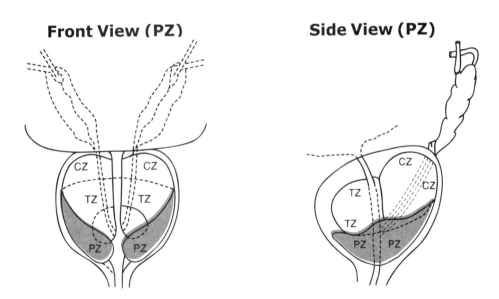

FIGURE F-2.—The Peripheral Zone (PZ) comprises 65–70% of the total area of the prostate (the largest zone of the prostate). Seventy percent of the cancers begin here. Most biopsy samples are taken from here.

The Central Zone

The central zone (CZ), the second-largest zone, is a cone-shaped region that makes up the majority of the base and much of the central portion of the prostate. It surrounds the ejaculatory ducts, where sperm from the testicles and fluid from the seminal vesicles meet to flow into the urethra. About 5% to 10% of prostate cancers begin growing in this zone, which cannot be examined during a DRE.

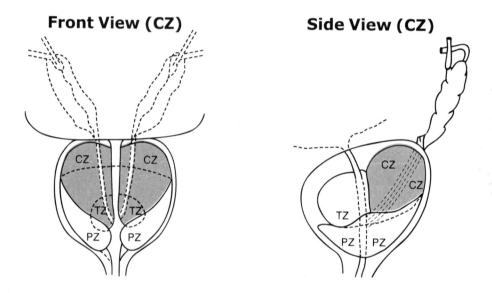

FIGURE F-3.—The Central Zone (CZ) comprises 20–25% of the total area of the prostate (the second largest zone of the prostate). Five to ten percent of the cancers begin here. A DRE cannot feel this area and a biopsy sample is usually not taken from here.

The Transition Zone

The transition zone (TZ) is the smallest of the three zones. It has two equal-sized lobes, one on each side of the prostatic urethra. This is sometimes called the BPH zone, because benign prostate hyperplasia, or noncancerous enlargement of the prostate, occurs only in this zone. Since this zone surrounds the urethra, BPH can cause many problems with urinary flow. About 15% to 20% of prostate cancers begin in the transition zone,

Front View (TZ)

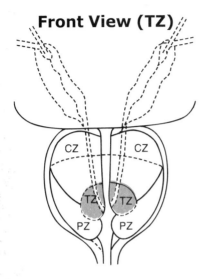

Side View (TZ)

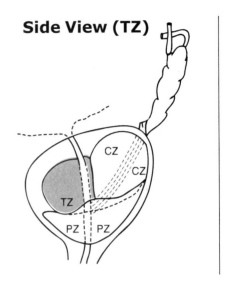

FIGURE F-4.—The Transition Zone (TZ) comprises 5–10% of the area of the total prostate. About 15–20% of the cancers begin here and BPH occurs here. A DRE cannot feel this area, but sometimes part of the biopsy sample is taken from here.

which cannot be reached during a DRE. However, since a number of cancers begin growing here, some physicians take biopsies from this area, as well as from the peripheral zone.

▶ The Prostatic Capsule

The prostatic capsule is the outer portion of the prostate. The capsule is significant in advanced prostate cancer because if it has been penetrated by the tumor, there is a greater possibility that the disease has or will spread beyond the prostate. If the capsule does not have signs of cancer, there is a good chance that it is still confined to the prostate.

▶ Apical Margin and Basilar or Bladder Neck Margin

The apical margin (near the apex) is the part of the prostate capsule that is near the bottom of the prostate, close to the urethra where it leaves the prostate. The basilar or bladder neck margin is the part of the capsule that is close to the top of the prostate and near the bladder.

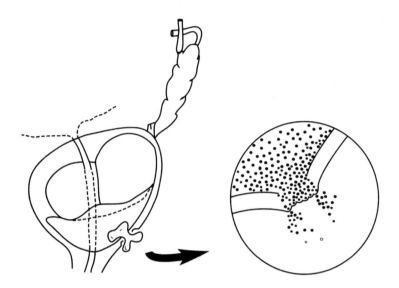

FIGURE F-5.—The Capsule of the prostate and Capsular Penetration by a cancer.

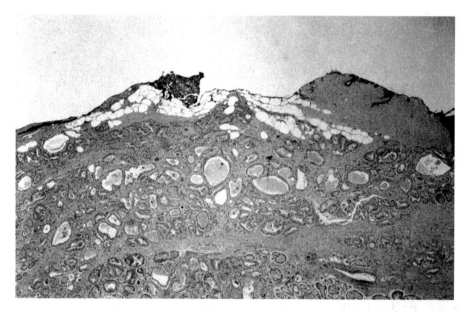

FIGURE F-6.—Cancer still within the margins of the prostate.

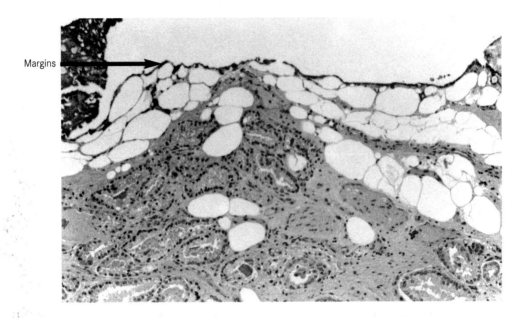

Margins

FIGURE F-7.—A closer look at a cancer still within the margins of the prostate.

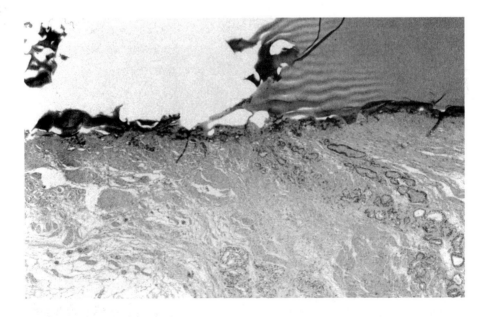

FIGURE F-8.—Cancer that has spread outside the margins of the prostate.

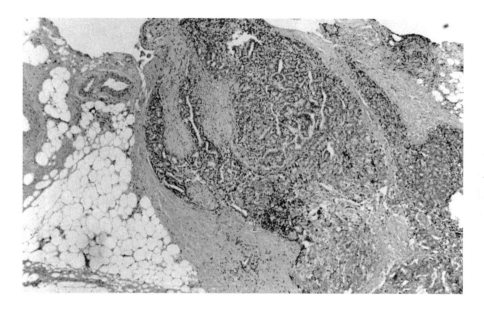

FIGURE F-9.—A closer look at cancer that has spread outside the margins of the prostate.

It is important to know about these two areas because if cancer is found in the apical margin after a radical prostatectomy, it may not be very significant—in other words, it does not necessarily mean that the cancer will move to adjacent areas. However, if there is cancer in the basilar or bladder neck margin, there is an increased possibility that the cancer has spread outside of the prostate.

▶ Neurovascular Bundles and Perineural Invasion

The neurovascular bundles are lengths of nerves, one on the left side of the prostate and one on the right, located near the rectum. These nerve bundles are very tiny, and difficult to find with the naked eye. Each carries nerves and blood to the penis to assist in achieving an erection. Years ago, before the discovery of these bundles, a radical prostatectomy often damaged them, causing most men to become impotent. Even if one or both of the bundles is spared during surgery, it does not guarantee that the man will be able to have natural erections—but it does increase the probability, especially if the man is younger. In some cases, the surgeon may not be able to spare these bundles because they have cancer or because they may allow the cancer easier access to other parts of the body. It all depends on where the cancer is located at the time of surgery. The term "perineural invasion" means that the cancer has invaded one or both bundles or the area around them.

▶ Dorsal Vein Complex

Blood is drained from the prostate by a number of veins, which together are called the "dorsal vein complex." When removing the prostate, surgeons have to be careful not to nick these veins because they carry a large amount of blood.

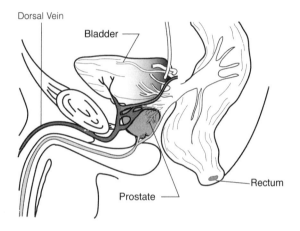

FIGURE F-10.—The Dorsal Vein Complex of the prostate.

▶ Seminal Vesicles

The seminal vesicles play a large role in advanced prostate cancer. There are two seminal vesicles located behind the bladder that drain into the urethra inside the prostate. Prostate cancer will often spread to the seminal vesicles, so they are typically removed during prostate surgery. The seminal vesicles make seminal fluid, which mixes with sperm from the testicles to make semen—the substance released from the penis during ejaculation. After prostate surgery, a man usually has "dry" orgasms because of the removal of the seminal vesicles.

▶ Testicles and Vas Deferens

The testicles make the hormone testosterone as well as sperm cells, which are transported by tubes (one from each testicle) that drain into the urethra. The ends of these tubes are called the "vas deferens," and they join the seminal vesicles, allowing sperm and seminal fluid to mix. The vas deferens lie close to the prostate and are vulnerable to spreading cancer, so both vas deferens are removed during a radical prostatectomy. This is why most men cannot father children after surgery. However, viable sperm can be extracted from the testicles after prostate surgery if a couple wants to have a baby.

The vas deferens is the part of the body that is cut and clamped during a vasectomy. However, in both prostate surgery and a vasectomy, the doctor is not removing the source of the sperm, just the path it takes. Sometimes small amounts of sperm will still find their

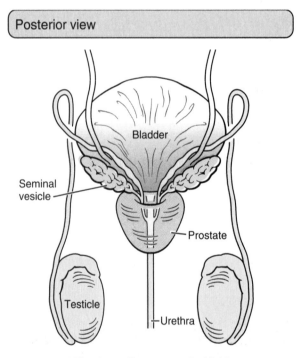

Ejaculate = Sperm + seminal fluid

FIGURE F-11.—Semen is sperm plus seminal fluid. Normal semen color is white and a normal sperm count is 100 million sperm cells per millimeter of semen. Testicles make sperm cells. The seminal vesicles make 60% of the seminal fluid and are a common place where cancer can go (they are removed during surgery).

way to the urethra. This only happens in a very small number of cases, but it means that a vasectomy or prostate surgery cannot provide a 100% guarantee that a man will never father a baby naturally again.

▶ ## The Urethra, the Bladder, and the Ureters

The urethra carries both sperm and urine to the tip of the penis. It begins at the bottom of the bladder and goes through the prostate at an angle, and then leaves the prostate and travels to and through the penis. The bladder stores urine until releasing it through the urethra during urination. The urine comes from the kidneys to the bladder by two tubes— the ureters. The bladder is especially significant in prostate cancer as cancer can spread there.

▶ ## The Internal and External Sphincters

A sphincter acts as a kind of door, opening and closing a part of the body. The area around the prostate has two sphincters of importance. First, there is the internal sphincter, which is located at the bottom of the bladder next to the point where the urethra begins. This internal sphincter is under "involuntary control," meaning that when the bladder is full, it may open without someone thinking about it. The internal sphincter also closes automatically when a man has an orgasm so that urine from the bladder does not mix with sperm from the testicles.

The external sphincter is located at the bottom (apex) of the prostate where the urethra leaves the prostate. This sphincter is under voluntary control and allows a man to hold his urine even if his bladder is ready to be emptied.

During a radical prostatectomy, radiation therapy, or other therapies, the internal sphincter might be partially removed or damaged. In most cases, however, the external sphincter will still holdback urine. However, both of these sites can be invaded by cancer from the prostate, and may have to be removed. Cancer can also damage these sphincters. As result, some men who have had prostate treatment or who have advanced prostate cancer suffer from incontinence, or the lack of urinary control. There are techniques that can be used to control incontinence, such as an artificial sphincter or collagen injections at the site of the internal sphincter.

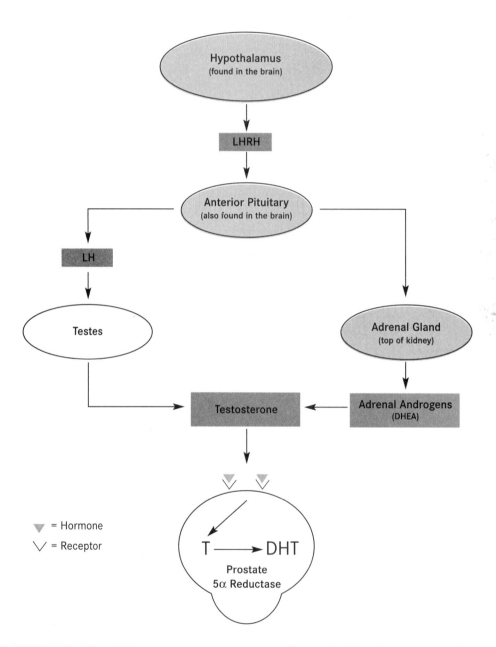

FIGURE F-12.—How testosterone is made and what happens when it gets into the prostate.

▶ **Denonvilliers' Fascia**

Denonvilliers' Fascia is named for Charles Pierre Denonvilliers, the French surgeon who discovered it in the 1800s. Denonvilliers' fascia is a piece of tissue located behind the prostate, separating the prostate from the rectum. Many surgeons remove this fascia when they are doing a radical prostatectomy, because it is an area often invaded by prostate cancer.

▶ **Lymph Nodes**

The body has a complex network of lymph vessels that transport protein, fat, excess fluid, and other materials. At various points along these vessels are pea-sized lymph nodes, which contain disease-fighting cells. Normally, these nodes are small, but if the body is fighting an infection, they can become enlarged, which is why a doctor might feel the nodes in the neck when someone has a sore throat.

There are lymph nodes near the prostate, but they cannot be felt with a finger because they lie deep within the body. However, they can be seen during surgery or with an imaging test. If cancer cells are present in the prostate area, these nodes may get larger as they fight the disease. In general, the greater the amount of cancer in the node, the larger the node may become. This is the basis of part of a prostate cancer staging system, which uses lymph nodes to gauge the seriousness of the cancer.

During prostate surgery, tissue from these nodes can be removed and then examined by a pathologist to determine whether or not the cancer has spread. The pathologist will report either "node positive" (+), meaning cancer was found in the nodes, or node negative (-), meaning no cancer was found in the nodes. Doctors may also refer to the number of nodes affected by cancer as "2 out of 10," or "1 out of 4," etc. The larger the number of nodes affected, the more the cancer has spread.

FINDING PROSTATE CANCER: PSA, FREE-PSA—PERCENT-FREE PSA, AND DRE TESTS

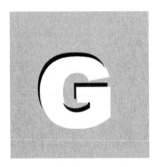

WHAT IS A PSA (PROSTATE-SPECIFIC ANTIGEN) TEST?

PROSTATE-SPECIFIC ANTIGEN (PSA) IS AN ENZYME PRODUCED BY THE PROSTATE. LARGE QUANTITIES OF PSA ARE FOUND IN SEMEN, WHICH IS RELEASED DURING EJACULATION, OR ORGASM. IN YOUNGER MEN, PSA IS NOT NORMALLY PRESENT IN THE BLOOD-STREAM IN LARGE AMOUNTS. HOWEVER, BECAUSE THE PROSTATE GLAND ENLARGES WITH AGE, IT IS NORMAL FOR OLDER MEN TO HAVE SLIGHTLY MORE PSA IN THEIR BLOOD BECAUSE THEIR PROSTATES PRODUCE MORE OF THIS ENZYME.

In addition to age-related prostate enlargement (a condition called benign prostatic hyperplasia, or BPH), another noncancerous condition that can cause PSA levels to rise is prostatitis, or infection and inflammation of the prostate. While BPH and prostatitis can elevate PSA levels, prostate cancer usually causes a more dramatic rise. However, about one in four prostate cancers do not cause an elevation in PSA. This is why the PSA blood test is not perfect and is part of the reason why its use has been controversial.

The PSA blood test is simple. One vial of blood is withdrawn, and sent to a laboratory. The result is usually reported within 24 hours.

The normal range for PSA in the bloodstream is 0–4 ng/ml (nanogram per milliliter). When a reading falls between 4–10 ng/ml, interpretation can become difficult. A result within this so-called "gray zone" could be normal for that individual or could indicate a variety of conditions, including cancer. This range varies according to age and race. For example, because the prostate enlarges with age, it is normal for the gland to secrete more PSA as a man gets older. If the PSA level goes beyond 4 ng/ml, however, this means that prostate cancer could be present, even though the doctor may not have felt anything suspicious during the DRE. This is why a prostate checkup should always include a DRE and a PSA blood test, because when used together, the chance of finding prostate cancer is much higher. In addition, some doctors also use the ultrasound test to detect prostate cancer, but it is not as reliable and accurate as the combination of DRE and PSA blood test.

Regardless of age and race, however, PSA levels greater than 10 ng/ml are a pretty accurate sign of prostate cancer; research shows that 70% to 80% of men with a result that high (also with a positive DRE) are found to have prostate cancer. But even if the numbers are frightening, a PSA test, alone or in combination with a DRE, only indicates there might be a problem; a prostate biopsy is always needed to confirm the presence of cancer.

Based on the data available today, the PSA test should be a part of the prostate checkup because it detects twice as many cancers as the DRE. Many of these are curable cancers that are still confined to the prostate. Everyone has a right to request the PSA test or to find another doctor who will request one. The American Cancer Society, the American Urological Association, and the American College of Radiology recommend the PSA test as part of the annual checkup for prostate cancer.

The PSA assay by itself, just like any other blood test, is not perfect. As a result, researchers are looking into new methods of interpreting PSA values to improve the test's accuracy. They are:

Age-Specific Reference Ranges

The discovery that PSA levels tend to rise with age has led to the use of "age-specific reference ranges" for determining normal PSA levels. Age-specific references ranges have increased the detection of prostate cancers in younger men (those under 60) and eliminated prostate biopsies in older men (those over 60), making PSA a more accurate and clinically useful test for diagnosing prostate cancer.

PSA Reference Ranges

Age Range	Asians	Blacks	Whites
40-49	0-2.0	0-2.0	0-2.5
50-59	0-3.0	0-4.0	0-3.5
60-69	0-4.0	0-4.5	0-4.5
70-79	0-5.0	0-5.5	0-6.5

PSA Density

(PSAD). A measurement technique in which the concentration of PSA in the blood is divided by the volume, or size, of the prostate gland, as measured by transrectal ultrasound. If this number, called PSA density, is greater than 0.15 and the PSA value is between 4–10 ng/ml, then a prostate biopsy is recommended. However, the use of PSA density in prostate-cancer screening is questionable. Many doctors who use age-specific PSA reference ranges do not bother to calculate the PSA density because they feel it is of no extra benefit. In general, the age-specific ranges provide as much information as PSA density and eliminate the need for a transrectal ultrasound.

PSA Velocity

(also called PSAV and PSA slope). This is an interpretation method that takes into account the change in PSA level over time. The currently accepted normal annual PSA level increase is a maximum of 0.75 ng/ml; an increase above this value could indicate cancer and an increase below this value could point toward BPH or a normal prostate. However, for PSA velocity to be a clinically useful tool, a man must have his blood tested for PSA at least three times over a period of at least two years. This gives a good overall picture of PSA production. PSA velocity is particularly useful in monitoring two types of men:

1. An individual whose PSA level is increasing rapidly but is still within the normal range (for example, if a 62-year-old man's PSA increased from 1.1 to 3.4 ng/ml in two years, his doctor may order a biopsy, even though the overall PSA level is still normal for his age).

2. An individuals with an elevated PSA level who has normal biopsy results (for example, if a patient has a PSA of 8.2 ng/ml but has a negative biopsy, the doctor can use PSA velocity to help determine whether a second biopsy will be necessary the following year. If the PSA level increases to 8.5 ng/ml, the doctor may not choose to biopsy again. If it rises to 9.6 ng/ml, however, a biopsy may be needed).

Studies have shown that PSA velocity is useful in reducing the number of unnecessary prostate biopsies. In men with BPH, for example, PSA velocity has reduced the number of biopsies from 4 in 10 to 1 in 10.

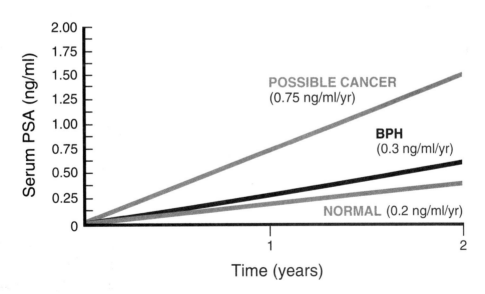

FIGURE G-1.—PSA velocity (the change in the PSA level over time) for men with cancer, benign prostatic hyperplasia and a normal prostate.

▶ Free PSA—Percent-Free PSA

There is plenty of ongoing research to find a better prostate-tumor marker or one that can be used in addition to the PSA test. However, in the future, there is one test that will be the focus of a lot of attention—the "percent-free" PSA test. This test will help to distinguish men with early prostate cancer from those who have an enlarged prostate gland. This test is currently being used experimentally at institutions around the country, and the

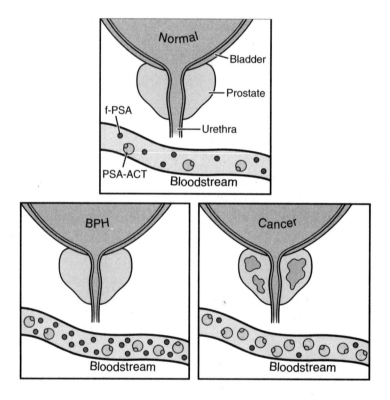

FIGURE G-2.—"Free" and "Complexed" molecular forms of PSA are deposited in the bloodstream in varying amounts, depending on the condition of the prostate. This is the basis of the new "Percent-Free PSA Test." At the top is a normal prostate, which releases small amounts of both Free (f-PSA) and Complexed PSA (PSA-ACT) into the bloodstream. At lower left is an enlarged, BPH-affected prostate, which typically releases higher amounts of Free PSA than normal. At the lower right is a cancerous prostate, which usually releases more complexed PSA than normal.

results are very encouraging. Men who have a PSA value in the gray zone (3–10 ng/ml) could have BPH or cancer, and they are good candidates for this new test, which looks at the various types of PSA that are produced by the prostate. In fact, the prostate produces at least six different types of PSA, two of which are found in large quantities in the bloodstream.

There is a "free" form and a "complexed" form of PSA. The current PSA blood test measures the total amount of free and complexed PSA to give a single PSA value. The new percent-free PSA test measures the quantity of free PSA and compares it to the total amount of PSA, both free and complexed. Research from Scandinavia has shown that measuring the proportion of free to total PSA can give the physician a better idea of whether the patient has BPH or prostate cancer. Men with BPH have higher amounts of free PSA, whereas men with prostate cancer have higher amounts of the complexed form.

Once the new test is widely adopted, future PSA exams will result in two separate scores: one will represent the total PSA level (free plus complexed PSA), which is the current standard; the other will represent the ratio of free to total PSA (percent-free PSA). Together the scores may significantly improve the diagnosis of prostate cancer.

Because the amount of complexed PSA increases with cancer, the ratio of free to total PSA is smaller in men with prostate cancer. For example, if a man without prostate cancer has a free-PSA level of 2 and a total-PSA level of 4, his percent-free PSA ratio would be 0.5 (2/4 = 0.5). On the other hand, if a man with prostate cancer has a free-PSA level of 2 and a total-PSA level of 8, his percent-free PSA ratio would be 0.25 (2/8 = 0.25). This lower ratio reflects an increase in complexed PSA, which is a likely indication of prostate cancer.

▶ Why is Screening with PSA Controversial?

Although the PSA blood test can detect prostate cancer while it is still curable and can reduce the number of needless biopsies in men with benign prostate enlargement, its use remains controversial for a variety of reasons.

Common arguments against using the PSA blood test:

- ▶ There has been no long-term, properly designed research study to show that early detection and subsequent treatment saves lives.

MOLECULAR FORMS OF PSA		
Forms of PSA	**Description**	**Detected by the PSA Test**
Free-PSA (f-PSA)	PSA not attached to anything (5% to 40% of the PSA in the blood that is detected by a PSA test	Yes
Complexed PSA (PSA-ACT)	PSA attached to a protein (65% to 90% of the PSA that is detected by a PSA test)	Yes
Total PSA (t-PSA)	All the PSA forms in the blood that are detected by a PSA test are made up of f-PSA and PSA-ACT	Yes
PSA-MG (also called) "occult PSA" or "hidden PSA"	PSA completely surrounded by a protein so it is not detectable by the PSA test	No
PSA-AT	Only very small amount found in the blood	No
PSA-ITI	Only very small amount found in the blood	No
PSA-PCI	Only found in the semen	No

▶ It may detect some cancers that are not "clinically significant," meaning that the tumor may be so small and grow so slowly that it might not be a threat to a man's life in the long run.

▶ It can give false-positive results, which means that some people may be led to believe they have prostate cancer when they do not, which creates a lot of anxiety for the man and unnecessary additional testing.

▶ Widespread use of the PSA test is expensive.

Common arguments in favor of the PSA blood test:

▶ There has been no long-term, properly designed research study to show that early detection and treatment does not save lives.

▶ Studies have shown that at least 85% of the prostate cancers being treated are clinically significant, that is, potentially life-threatening.

▶ It can detect prostate cancers at a more localized, early stage while they are still curable. However, the PSA test must be used along with the DRE to ensure the most accurate results.

▶ What Factors Could Affect the PSA Level?

Just because a PSA level is high or has increased does not necessarily mean someone has prostate cancer. There are two common, noncancerous causes of PSA elevation: age-related enlargement of the prostate, or BPH; and prostatitis, or infection of the prostate gland. Below is a list of other conditions, medical procedures, and medications that can trigger temporary changes in PSA levels.

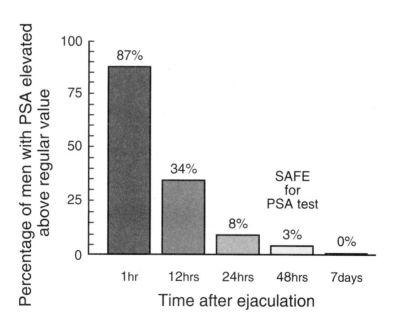

FIGURE G-3.—After ejaculation, most men experience an increase in their PSA that can be large enough to falsely suggest the presence of cancer. However, after about 48 hours, the PSA level typically returns to normal.

Conditions

Acute urinary retention. This condition, in which urination becomes impossible, is often associated with severe enlargement of the prostate. Emergency medical intervention is required.

Ejaculation. Among men 50–79 years of age, PSA levels rise significantly after ejaculation (orgasm). PSA levels increase up to 40% within an hour of ejaculation and return to normal within 48 hours. Therefore, men age 50 and older should refrain from ejaculation for at least two days before undergoing a PSA test to ensure the most accurate results. Men in this age group can experience higher PSA levels after ejaculation because the tissue barriers that keep the enzyme within the prostate, where it is manufactured, deteriorate with age; thus, older prostates can be more "leaky" than younger prostates. When a man ejaculates, the muscle of the prostate contracts and relaxes, which basically "massages" the gland. Among men in their 50s, 60s, and 70s, this activity can allow PSA to escape more easily into the bloodstream.

Medical Procedures

All of the following urological procedures cause a temporary elevation in the PSA level:

▶ Balloon dilation of the prostate
▶ High-intensity focused ultrasound (HIFU)
▶ Transrectal ultrasound (TRUS)-guided biopsy
▶ Transurethral incision of the prostate (TUIP)
▶ Transurethral microwave therapy (TUMT)
▶ Transurethral needle ablation (TUNA)
▶ Transurethral resection of the prostate (TURP)
▶ Visual laser ablation of the prostate (VLAP)

After undergoing a prostate biopsy or any of the above treatments for benign prostatic enlargement, a man should wait at least six weeks for the PSA level to return to baseline, or normal, before scheduling a cancer-screening test.

Medications

Finasteride (trade name Proscar®). This FDA-approved drug for benign prostatic hyperplasia (BPH) helps shrink the prostate and may reduce its symptoms. It can also reduce the PSA level by 50%. Thus, someone taking Proscar whose doctor uses age-specific reference ranges for the PSA blood test, would find their result cut in half. For example, for a 75-year-old white male who has a normal PSA reference range of 0–6.5 ng/ml, taking Proscar would reduce his range to 0–3.25 ng/ml. **Dutasteride** is a new drug that has some similar characteristics to Finasteride, but it may reduce DHT levels to a greater degree. Talk with your doctor about both these medications.

▶ Are all PSA Tests Created Equal?

There are six FDA-approved PSA blood tests, or assays, on the market in the United States; more than 30 are being used in Europe. However, not all of these tests are exactly the same. Therefore, PSA results can vary slightly, depending on which brand of test is used and which laboratory analyzes the test. The results of PSA tests performed on the same individual even hours or minutes apart can vary up to 8%, regardless of whether the same brand of test is used. These changes are not considered significant enough to be of concern, but to ensure the most consistent results, an annual PSA test should be processed by the same laboratory each time. If this is not possible, then at least request that the same brand of test be used consistently.

▶ PSA and Advanced Disease

Since 1992, the PSA blood test has been used to measure the response of advanced prostate cancer to various treatments. Several studies and trials have shown a direct relationship between decreases in PSA and shrinkage of measurable prostate tumors as well as increased survival rates for men who decreased their PSA level by greater than 50% from their baseline value.

A special note on the use of PSA and advanced prostate cancer: In localized disease, a PSA of 4 can be used as an upper limit of normal to screen for cancer, but this is not the case with androgen-independent cancers. Each tumor creates a unique amount of PSA, which is relative to each individual. Thus, each individual has a unique starting point, or baseline; someone may have a small amount of cancer and a high PSA, or a large amount of cancer and a low PSA.

It is essentially meaningless to compare one person's PSA level with that of someone else. There are men who have a PSA of less than 10 who have many bone metastases and need narcotics to control their pain. Other men with PSAs over 1,000 have no pain. There is no specific PSA value that correlates with symptoms or death.

What is a Digital Rectal Exam?

During a digital rectal (DRE) exam, the doctor's gloved and lubricated index finger (digit) is inserted into the rectum to feel for any suspicious changes on the surface of the prostate. The index finger is used because it is the most sensitive finger on the hand. The

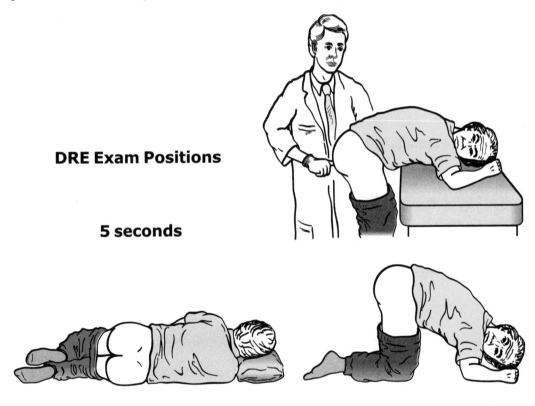

DRE Exam Positions

5 seconds

FIGURE G-4.—The Digital-Rectal Prostate Examination (DRE) itself takes about five seconds and can be performed at least three different ways: by having the patient stand and lean over the examining table (top right); by having the patient lie on his side, curled into a fetal position on top of the examining table (lower left); or by having the the patient kneel face-down on top of the examination table (lower right).

rectum is thin and flexible enough so that the prostate can be easily felt, much like a golf ball through a piece of wax paper. The doctor usually inserts about one-half the finger to feel the gland, but this depends on the man's weight. In a heavier man, more of the finger may be inserted.

The DRE is simple to perform. The doctor will ask the man to put on a hospital robe/ gown or to drop his pants. The man will be asked to assume a position, which position depends on the doctor. The man may be asked to: (1) stand next to the examining table and to bend forward a little; (2) kneel on the examining table; or (3) lie on his side (in a fetal position). All of these positions make it easier for the doctor's finger to travel through the anus and into the rectum so the prostate can be felt.

The DRE itself is very quick, generally less than a minute in length. It may feel strange, but it should not be painful. If it is painful, the doctor should be told, because it could be a sign of a prostate disorder such as prostatitis, or inflammation of the prostate.

The exam is also safe; if performed correctly, there is little to no chance of rectal injury. It also costs very little—just the price of a latex glove, some lubricant, and a small amount of the doctor's time.

The DRE is necessary because most prostate cancers begin in the PZ, which can only be felt through this type of exam. Therefore, the DRE can detect localized cancer—cancer that has not spread beyond the prostate—and current treatments can potentially cure this type of cancer.

The doctor that performs the DRE has probably performed hundreds or even thousands of these tests. This is a routine exam that could easily prevent an early death.

OTHER TESTS
RELATED TO DETECTING
AND UNDERSTANDING
PROSTATE CANCER

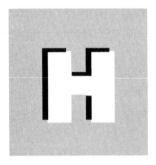

There are many ways to diagnose and analyze prostate cancer, both when it is localized as well as when it has spread outside the prostate (advanced cancer). Currently, the only "official" way to diagnose prostate cancer is through a biopsy. Depending on the situation, a man may or may not have one or more of these tests done.

▶ Alkaline Phosphatase

The alkaline phosphatase test is a simple blood test. Alkaline phosphatase is an enzyme made in the liver, bones, kidneys, intestines, and placenta. The body produces more of it when the liver and/or bones are being damaged. The test result gives the doctor a sense of the rate of liver and/or bone damage being caused by prostate cancer. This test is usually done on someone suspected of having advanced disease that has spread to the liver and/or bones.

▶ Angiogenesis ~ (also called)
"Microvessel Density" or MVD and "Neovascularity"

An angiogenesis test is performed on the pathology biopsy. If an area of the body is not getting enough blood, the affected tissue may respond by releasing certain substances that cause blood vessels to grow toward in a process called angiogenesis. It occurs during pregnancy to supply blood to the fetus, or when a wound or tissue is trying to recover from an injury. It can also happen in abnormal tissues such as cancer. Some researchers think that by assessing the blood vessels in tissue samples, doctors will be able to tell how far a cancer has spread, and perhaps predict how a cancer may act. In the angiogenesis test, a pathologist examines tissue removed during surgery or biopsy. The tissue sample is stained to make blood vessels more visible, and the blood vessels are counted, either manually or by a computer. It is not known at this time how much practical value this test will be and it is considered experimental.

▶ Biopsy of the Prostate ~ (also called)
Transrectal Ultrasound-guided Biopsy

A prostate biopsy is the best way to determine whether or not cancer exists in the prostate. It can be very helpful in determining whether cancer has spread beyond the prostate. A pathologist can look at the biopsy sample to see if the capsule of the prostate has been penetrated by the cancer, and at tissue from around the prostate to look for signs of locally-advanced disease. In general, a biopsy is appropriate when there is a good possibility of someone having cancer, based on a positive DRE, an elevated PSA level, and/or a suspicious site on an ultrasound.

A biopsy involves taking a small sample of tissue that is examined by a pathologist to determine whether or not it is cancerous. An ultrasound probe is inserted into the rectum so that a physician can view the prostate on an ultrasound machine. The probe has a small biopsy needle that can go through the lining of the rectum and into the prostate so that a small piece of tissue (also called a "core") can be removed and examined. While this procedure is uncomfortable, it is brief (a few minutes) and medication can be given so the procedure is easier to tolerate.

There are two types of biopsy needles: a 14-gauge needle and a newer, smaller 18-gauge needle. The 18-gauge needle has some advantages, including a reduced chance of post-biopsy infection, a better chance of getting a quality sample, less discomfort, and a decrease in the false negative rate (that is, if no cancer is found there is a good chance that no cancer is actually there). The disadvantage is that it provides a smaller sample for examination than the 14-gauge needle.

There is some question about how many biopsy samples should be taken at one time. Currently, most doctors take what is called a "sextant" biopsy, which means six pieces of tissue are taken from different areas of the PZ of the prostate. Some doctors may take less and some may take more. For example, some physicians take eight biopsy samples at one

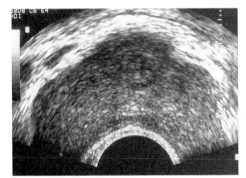
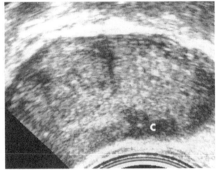

Normal (negative)   **Abnormal (positive);**
"C" represents cancer

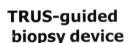

TRUS-guided
biopsy device

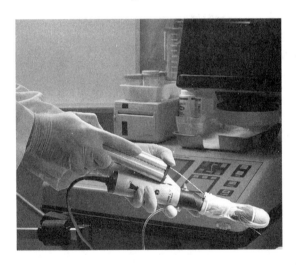

FIGURE H-1.—The Transrectal Ultrasound (TRUS)-guided biopsy device (bottom), and examples of a normal and abnormal prostate ultrasound (top left and right).

Normal

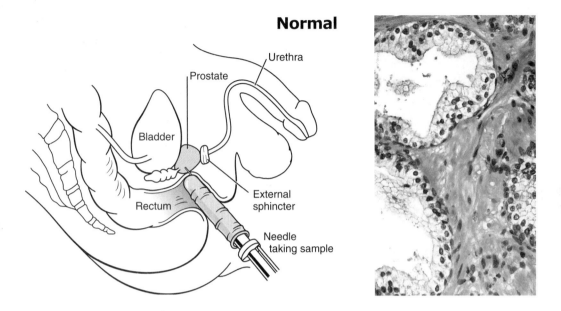

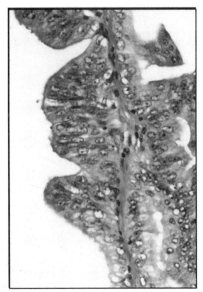

Cancerous

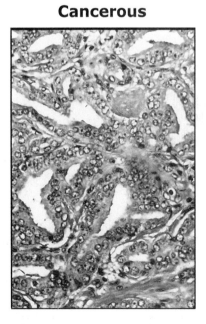

PIN "gray zone"

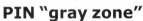

FIGURE H-2.—The Prostate Biopsy procedure itself (top left) and the three types of prostate cells that can be found: normal, "gray zone" (PIN), or cancerous.

time, six from the PZ and two from the TZ. And, if the physician suspects that cancer has spread to the seminal vesicles, a biopsy(s) may also be taken from there.

Ask the physician how many biopsies will be taken and from what parts of the prostate. There is a basic tradeoff: The fewer samples taken, the less likely it is that someone may experience complications, such as bleeding or infection, from the biopsy, but the chances of missing cancerous tissue increase. The more biopsies taken, the more likely it is that someone will experience complications, but there is also a higher likelihood of finding any cancer that is present.

▶ Bone Scan ~ (also called)
"Radionuclide Bone Scan" or "Radioisotopic Bone Scan"

A bone scan shows whether or not cancer has spread to any of the bones. It is an imaging test that lets doctors take a "picture" of the skeleton. Before the procedure, a harmless dye or isotope—typically called Technetium—is injected into a vein. Approximately three hours later an X-ray machine is passed around the body and films are taken. This is a painless procedure with the exception of the initial dye injection. The dye travels throughout the body and becomes concentrated in areas of the skeleton or bone that may have cancer—areas that are sometimes referred to as "hot spots." Hot spots can occur because of an old injury, arthritis, infection in the bone, or because of cancer. For example, if a hot spot appears on both sides of the body in the same location, it is usually not an indication of cancer. For example, if there is a spot on the 4th right rib and a spot on the 4th left rib at the same location, then it is probably not cancerous. More likely, it represents arthritis or some other disease. However, if a dark spot appears on the 4th right rib and there is nothing on the left rib, then the hot spot is more likely to indicate the presence of cancer.

This is a good test for anyone suspected of having advanced prostate cancer. It should be performed if someone has any or all of the following:

- ▶ Bone pain after being diagnosed with prostate cancer.
- ▶ Clinical evidence of advanced disease.
- ▶ High alkaline phosphatase level (sometimes).
- ▶ High Gleason score (8 – 10) at diagnosis.
- ▶ PSA level greater than 10 at diagnosis.

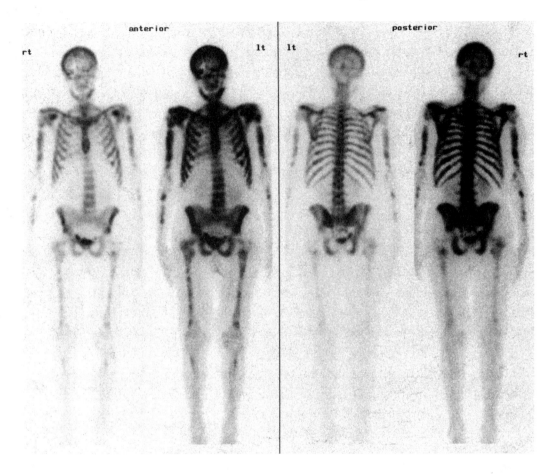

FIGURE H-3.—Bone Scan from an advanced prostate cancer patient.

Once a bone scan has been performed, it can be used as a basis for comparing and interpreting later bone scans, and identifying changes in the bones over time.

► Color Doppler Imaging "CDI" ~ (also called) Transrectal Color Doppler Imaging

Color Doppler imaging is an experimental form of ultrasound testing where an ultrasound probe is placed in the rectum and sound waves are used to produce an image of the prostate. While it is mildly uncomfortable, most men have no problem with the test. Cancer cells need blood, and as they grow, an abnormal flow of blood is often created around the cancer (see Angiogenesis). Scientists hope that by being able to detect that flow, they will also be able to detect the cancer it is supplying. That's where color Doppler imaging plays a part.

In the images, different colors correspond to the degree of blood flow to the cancer. Cancers that have little to no blood flow going to them are given a low number (such as 0 or +1), and cancers that have a lot of blood flowing to them are given higher number (+2 or above). This test is relatively new and is not widely used. It is uncertain how helpful it is going to be in the treatment of cancer.

▶ Computed Axial Tomography "CAT" Scan ~ (also called) CT Scan

A computed axial tomography (CAT) scan, commonly called a CT scan, is an X-ray imaging test, but is much more sensitive than an ordinary X-ray. The CT scan is used to look for the presence of cancer throughout the body, especially in lymph nodes and the liver. An iodine-based solution (a contrast material) is injected into an arm vein to help make the pictures clear. As the IV solution goes in, there may be a temporary rush of heat throughout the body, but it is not painful. People who are allergic to iodine can have the scan without the use of a contrast solution. The procedure takes 15 to 45 minutes. The scan produces detailed, cross-sectional images of the body. When these images are electronically stacked on top of each other and shown on a computer screen, the doctor may view a specific part of the body and its surrounding structures from every angle. This helps radiation oncologists with treatment planning.

▶ DNA Ploidy

The DNA Ploidy test is performed on the pathology specimen. It analyzes the DNA from cancer cells obtained in a biopsy or through surgery in order to help determine how aggressive the cancer might be. There are three types of DNA that can be found in cells:

- ▶ Diploid is the normal type of DNA.
- ▶ Aneuploid (also called nondiploid) is abnormal DNA—there is less or more DNA than normal.
- ▶ Tetraploid (also called nondiploid) is abnormal DNA—there is double or twice as much DNA as normal.

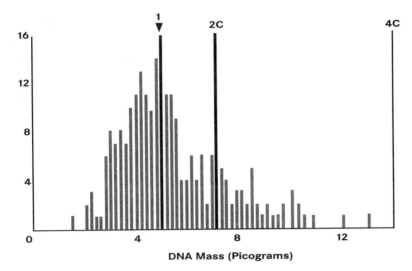

FIGURE H-4.—Distribution of DNA Mass.

There are three techniques used to test DNA ploidy: flow cytometry, static image analysis, and fluorescence in situ hybridization (FISH). These vary in technical detail, but all three strive to provide information that can help stage and grade cancer. For example, some men with diploid tumors have a greater chance of survival than those with aneuploid or tetraploid tumors.

At this point, DNA Ploidy tests are probably most appropriate for people with localized or locally-advanced cancer, when doctors want to get some idea of where the disease might go in the future. Some hospitals consider this a routine test and give this information as part of pathology reports. However, other doctors and hospitals still consider the test to be experimental.

▶ Hemoglobin (Hb)

The hemoglobin test is a blood test that is commonly done in the doctor's office. Hemoglobin is the molecule that carries oxygen in the blood. A low hemoglobin indicates anemia, and someone may become tired or fatigued easily and short of breath. Doctors working with prostate patients track hemoglobin because some treatments, such as chemotherapy, can lower hemoglobin levels. Low hemoglobin can be treated with a blood transfusion.

This test is usually done at the start of or during therapy that can lower hemoglobin levels, such as hormone ablation or chemotherapy. Some studies have suggested that the hemoglobin level can be used in predicting who will do well on a certain chemotherapy program, but this has not been proven.

▶ Insulin Growth Factor-1 (IGF-1)

Insulin growth factor-1 (IGF-1) is a growth factor. Growth factors are released by cells in the body to stimulate cell growth and development. Recent research has shown that men who have higher levels of IGF-1 in their bloodstream may be at an increased risk of being diagnosed with prostate cancer.

The level of IGF-1 is assessed through a blood test. In the future, people may have their IGF-1 level checked to see if they are at increased risk of getting cancer, in much the same way that cholesterol is checked today to gauge a person's risk for heart disease. Currently, this test is experimental and not available.

▶ Laparoscopic Pelvic Lymphadenectomy ~ (also called) Pelvic Lymph Node Dissection

When the lymph nodes are invaded by prostate cancer, they often do not become enlarged, making it hard to detect the spread of cancer through CT scans and other tests that look for increased size. As a result, doctors sometimes sample nodes for cancer, removing some tissue in a minor surgical procedure called laparoscopic pelvic lymphadenectomy, or pelvic lymph node dissection (PLND).

There are actually three types of PLND that can be done. These are all types of surgery with varying sizes of incisions. This procedure should be discussed with the urologist. The type of procedure used may depend on how many lymph nodes the urologist wants to examine.

- ▶ Open pelvic lymph node dissection
- ▶ Minilaparotomy for pelvic lymph node dissection (also called "minilap")
- ▶ Laparoscopic pelvic lymph node dissection

In the past, this was a common procedure to tell if prostate cancer had spread (called staging the cancer). As other tests have become better, these procedures are becoming less and less common.

▶ Lactate Dehydrogenase (LDH)

Lactate dehydrogenase (LDH) is a simple blood test. LDH is an enzyme found in the blood and many body organs. An LDH blood test is not a specific test for prostate cancer—it can also be used in monitoring people who are having a heart attack or who have liver disease. Some studies have suggested that LDH levels go up when someone's prostate cancer is more active. Therefore, some physicians use it to monitor a someone's response to chemotherapy. Others have suggested that LDH, like alkaline phosphatase and hemoglobin, may be useful in predicting the future course of some prostate cancers.

▶ Monoclonal Antibodies ~ (also called) Immunoscintigraphy "CYT-356" or ProstaScint® "7E11-5.3"

Monoclonal antibodies (also called immunoscintigraphy or CYT-356; ProstaScint®; or 7E11-C5.3) is a painless imaging test that involves an injection into the bloodstream of special antibodies with a radioactive imaging agent attached. These antibodies travel throughout the body and attach themselves to cancerous tissue. The concentrated antibodies show up on an image as dark areas when X-rays or scans are taken. Two imaging sessions are needed to get results. The first session involves the injection of the antibodies. About 30 minutes later, a number of pictures (scans) are taken. This procedure usually takes about an hour and provides baseline images for the test. Two to five days later the scans are repeated. This allows for the injected material to concentrate in areas where there may be cancer. The night before the second session, an oral laxative is taken. The next morning an enema is given and the bladder is emptied—all of which helps ensure clear images. This scanning session lasts two or three hours.

Monoclonal antibodies have generated a lot of interest in the past few years. They have been used for some time to find cancers of the colon, ovary, and lungs. In 1996, a monoclonal antibody called capromab pendetide (also called CP, and sold under the name ProstaScint®) received FDA approval for use in detecting prostate cancer.

Currently, this test is used mainly with men who:

▶ Have a newly diagnosed prostate cancer that is localized and may be at high risk for spread to the lymph nodes.

▶ Have undergone a radical prostatectomy or other curative procedure and are now experiencing a rising PSA with no detectable cancer recurrence through conventional imaging techniques such as CT scans or MRI.

The ProstaScint® scan may or may not be helpful. This is because it is a test that may be positive in areas where there is no cancer (not specific enough), and negative in areas where there really is cancer (not sensitive enough). At this point, it is not a routine test for prostate cancer staging, but is used when the doctor thinks it may be useful in helping decide which treatment is appropriate.

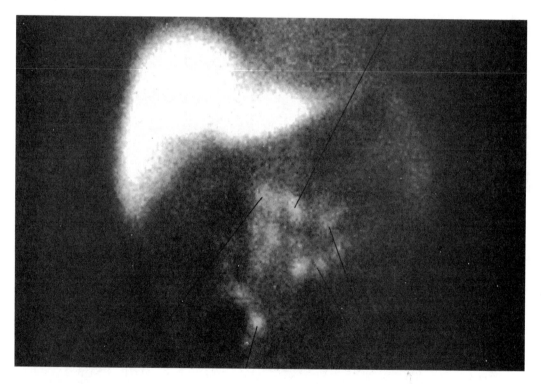

FIGURE H-5.—ProstaScint scan shows lighted areas, which means there may be some cancer in those lymph nodes (the large lighted area at the top of the picture is a normal liver with no cancer. It is lighted up because it usually absorbs a lot of the dye.

▶ Magnetic Resonance Imaging (MRI) and Endorectal Coil MRI

Magnetic resonance imaging (MRI) uses a magnetic field, rather than radiation, to produce images of the body. During the procedure, a series of images is created while the individual lies in an open tube for 30 to 45 minutes. There is also a new version of this test, called Endorectal Coil MRI, which uses a small probe inserted into the rectum to take pictures of the prostate and the areas around it.

The MRI offers no advantage over transrectal ultrasound (TRUS) tests in staging more localized cancers. In fact, TRUS has been found to be a better indicator of determining whether or not cancer has become locally advanced.

The Endorectal Coil MRI, on the other hand, has produced some interesting results lately. In a recent study, for men who had a moderately elevated PSA (10 – 20) and a moderate Gleason score (5 – 7), the test was able to determine whether the seminal vesicles had cancer more than 95% of the time. However, more studies are needed to see if this test can provide additional information beyond that which is currently available through PSA, Gleason scores, and other methods. The test is still experimental, but it is being used in many hospitals.

▶ Prostatic Acid Phosphatase (PAP)

The prostatic acid phosphatase (PAP) blood test, which is not related to the PAP smear used to test for abnormalities of the cervix, has actually been around for more than 50 years and was widely used before the PSA test was developed. The test determines the level of PAP, an enzyme of unknown function, thought to be a marker of prostate cancer, which is released by the prostate and present in the blood. It is fairly good at detecting advanced prostate cancer, but not at staging the disease. If the PAP level is elevated, it may point to the spread of cancer beyond the prostate. If the PAP is normal, it does not really tell much, because it could mean that cancer has spread beyond the prostate or is confined to the prostate. This test is rarely used, having been more or less replaced by the more accurate PSA test.

▶ Reverse Transcriptase-Polymerase Chain Reaction (RT-PCR)

Reverse transcriptase-polymerase chain reaction (RT-PCR) is usually a blood test, but in a small number of cases it can also be performed using bone marrow and/or lymph node samples. The RT-PCR looks for traces of PSA or prostate-specific membrane antigen (PSMA) in areas of the body that do not normally secrete PSA or PSMA. In other words, it looks for cancer cells that have left the prostate and spread to other parts of the body. This test is experimental, but in laboratories it has been able to detect the presence of just one prostate cell in a group of 1 million nonprostate cells. Unfortunately, doctors do not know what that means yet. Someone might be asked to give a sample of blood or bone marrow to undergo this test as part of an experimental trial.

▶ Transrectal Ultrasound (TRUS)

Transrectal ultrasound (TRUS) is a procedure that uses sound waves to detect the difference between cancerous and noncancerous prostate tissue. An ultrasound probe is placed inside the rectum, hence the name "transrectal" ultrasound. The ultrasound probe is used to produce a picture of the prostate and its surroundings so that a physician can view it on an ultrasound machine. While this procedure is uncomfortable, it is brief (a few minutes) and medication will help someone relax and tolerate the procedure with ease.

A prostate biopsy is performed under the guidance of TRUS, in which the sound waves from the rectal ultrasound probe act as a navigator to let the doctor accurately locate the prostate for tissue sampling. A tiny needle is then inserted alongside the probe to remove a small sample of prostate tissue, about 1/25th of an inch thick. Usually a minimum of six individual pieces of tissue (called a sextant biopsy) are taken from different areas around the PZ of the prostate (the area where three of every four cancers begin to grow). Some doctors also take two additional samples from the TZ of the prostate, which is where one in four prostate cancers begins. The biopsies are sent to a pathologist, which is a doctor who specializes in diagnosing cancer or other abnormalities from tissue samples.

Although there is some discomfort with this procedure, it provides a better picture of the prostate and the areas around it. TRUS can not only help doctors diagnose disease, it is also useful in staging prostate cancer and in finding locally-advanced disease.

▶ X-rays

X-rays are simple—and for most people, familiar—tests. X-rays play a fairly small role in diagnosing prostate cancer, being used primarily to determine whether a person's disease has spread to other parts of the body. They are not routinely used as part of the work-up in a man with newly diagnosed prostate cancer. However, they may be used to look at the lungs or bones to help decide if there is an infection or cancer present.

HOW AGGRESSIVE (GRADING) AND WHERE (STAGING) IS YOUR CANCER?

WHAT DOES THE CANCER LOOK LIKE UNDER THE MICROSCOPE (GRADING)?

A PROSTATE CANCER BIOPSY REMOVES VERY SMALL TISSUE SAMPLES THAT ARE SENT TO A PATHOLOGIST TO BE EXAMINED OR "GRADED." THIS INFORMATION TELLS JUST HOW AGGRESSIVE AND FAST-GROWING A CANCER MIGHT BE.

There are many grading systems used by doctors. These systems vary, of course, but they all provide some insight into the nature of the cancer by categorizing it with a grade. The higher the grade, the more the cancer cells do not look like normal cells—and therefore, the more aggressive the cancer and the more likely it is that it will grow and spread quickly. Conversely, the lower the grade, the more the cancer cells look like normal cells— and therefore, the less aggressive the cancer and the more likely it is that the disease will grow and spread slowly.

The most widely used grading system is the Gleason grading system. To determine a Gleason grade, a pathologist looks at the cancerous tissue sample and assigns it two numbers between 1 and 5. Two numbers are given because prostate tumors from a single

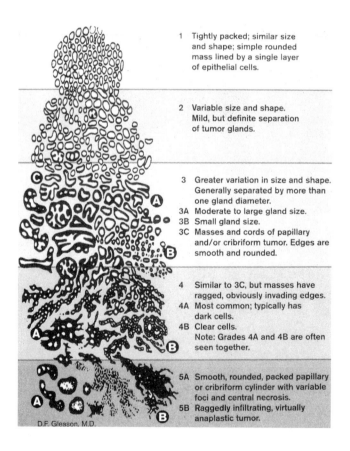

FIGURE I-1.—Prostatic Adenocarcinoma (Histologic Grades).

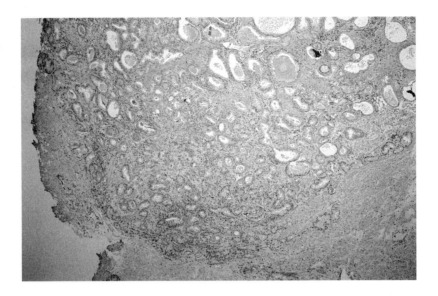

FIGURE I-2.—Gleason Grade 1.

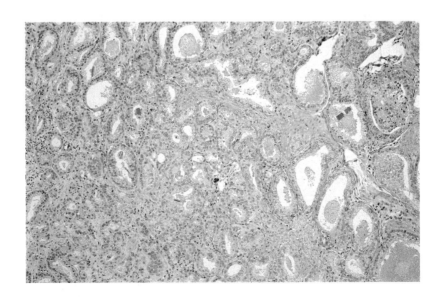

FIGURE I-3.—Gleason Grade 2.

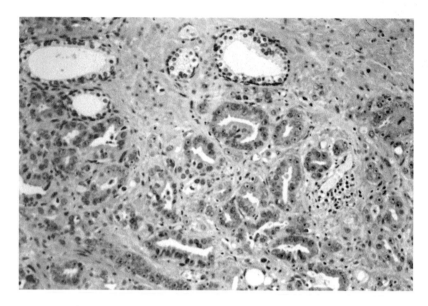

FIGURE I-4.—Gleason Grade 3.

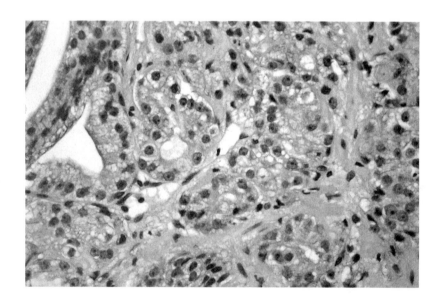

FIGURE I-5.—Gleason Grade 4.

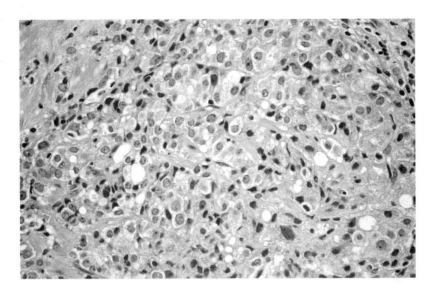

FIGURE I-6.—Gleason Grade 5.

individual will usually show some variation. In other words, some of the tumor might look aggressive, while some of it may not. The pathologist is concerned about the overall appearance of the tumor, and so uses the grades of the two most predominant types of tissue, and combines them to come up with a total score for the tumor. The first number is the most predominant type and the second number is the second most common type seen on the slides.

TABLE I-1.—Gleason Systems		
Older	**Newer**	**What Does It Mean?**
2–4	2–4	A well-differentiated cancer that looks a lot like normal prostate cells and is slightly aggressive
5–7	5–6	A moderately-differentiated cancer that looks somewhat like normal cells and is moderately aggressive
—	7	A moderately poorly-differentiated cancer that looks only a little like normal cells and is aggressive
8–10	8–10	A poorly-differentiated cancer that does not look anything like normal cells and is very aggressive

TABLE I-2.—Possible Gleason Scores	
Gleason Scores	**What Does that Tell Us?**
1+1, 2+1, 1+2, 1+3 2+1, 2+2 3+1	2–4 = Well differentiated cancer or not aggressive
1+4, 1+5 2+3, 2+4 3+2, 3+3 4+1, 4+2 5+1	5–6 = Moderately differentiated cancer or moderately aggressive
2+5 3+4 4+3 5+2	7 = Moderately poorly-differentiated or aggressive
3+5 4+4, 4+5 5+3, 5+4, 5+5	8–10 = Poorly differentiated cancer or very aggressive

A Gleason total score will be somewhere between 2 and 10, with scores between 2 and 4 being the least aggressive cancers, 5 through 7 being moderately aggressive, and 8 through 10 being very aggressive. A pathology report might say that a Gleason score is "3 + 4 = 7," which is the two individual scores and their total. Other reports might just say "3 + 4," or "7 total" or "7 overall." Be sure to ask for the full set of numbers—the total Gleason score and the two individual scores. Many doctors are beginning to think that it is only the most predominant type of cancer that is important for prognosis; that is, telling whether the cancer has already or may someday spread. For example, a 3 + 4 = 7 may be better to have than a 4 + 3 = 7 cancer. (Remember, the first number is the most predominant type and the second number is the second most common type seen on the slides.) However, it is still too early to know for sure if this is true.

The Gleason grading system has recently undergone a minor change, which has yet to be fully adopted by the medical community. In the newer version, there is a separate category for the number 7. In the older system, the Gleason number 7 was grouped with the numbers 5 and 6. This change was made because physicians noticed that cancers with Gleason scores of 7 did not look or act like those with scores of 5 and 6 or 8 and 10. So they have been given their own category.

Statistically, the following is what is currently known about the total Gleason scores and cancer:

► 2.1% of the Gleason scores of 2 – 4 spread beyond the prostate in a year if they are not treated. Therefore, in five years the chance of spread is about 10%; in 10 years, about 20% to 25%; in 15 years about 30% to 33%; and in 20 years about 40% to 45%. That is, of course, fairly slow growth—and not surprisingly, the majority of older men with localized cancer and a low Gleason score die of something other than prostate cancer, regardless of whether or not they have treatment.

► 5.4% of the Gleason scores of 5 – 7 will spread beyond the prostate in a year if they are not treated. Therefore, in five years the chance of spread is about 25% to 30%; in 10 years, about 50% to 55%; in 15 years about 80% to 85%; and in 20 years, about 100%.

► 13.5% of the Gleason scores of 8 – 10 will spread beyond the prostate in a year if they are not treated. Therefore, in five years the chance of spread is about 65% to 70%, and in 10 years, about 100%. Clearly, men with high Gleason scores have a much higher risk of getting advanced prostate cancer.

Do Gleason scores change over time? Research seems to indicate that they usually do not change that much—so a 5 today will probably mean a 5 tomorrow. However, doctors may change their minds about what the score is. Different pathologists may disagree on a Gleason score, or the biopsy may have revealed only part of the cancer, making the Gleason number inaccurate. In fact, about 25% of the Gleason scores are "undergraded," meaning the score is lower than it should be for the cancer in question. And about 25% of the Gleason scores are "overgraded," with a number that is higher than it should be. If someone is concerned about their Gleason score, have another pathologist review the tissue samples.

Men with prostate cancer should know their Gleason scores. A Gleason score gives the doctor an idea of how aggressive the cancer may be, which helps determine the kind of treatment needed.

▶ How Far Has the Cancer Spread (Staging)?

In addition to knowing how aggressive a man's prostate cancer is, doctors also want to determine how far it has spread, and where it is located. Making this determination is called "staging" the cancer.

There are two types of staging systems in use today: The ABCD system (also called the Whitmore-Jewett system), and the newer TNM staging system. Some doctors use one, some use the other, and some use both. Therefore, it is important to understand both systems.

The ABCD system uses those four letters to describe stages:

▶ **"A"** means the tumor is localized and was found during a procedure unrelated to cancer, such as a TURP, which is a surgery for the treatment of BPH.

▶ **"B"** means the tumor is still localized, but was found by DRE, PSA test, or some other method used to detect cancer.

▶ **"C"** means the tumor has left the prostate and may have reached other structures near the prostate.

▶ **"D"** means the tumor has spread far beyond the prostate to the lymph nodes, lungs, bone, or other organs.

A number from 0 to 2 is usually placed next to the letter. The higher the number, the more space the cancer takes up in that location or the farther it has spread. So, for example, a C2 cancer and a C1 cancer have both left the prostate, as indicated by the letter C, but the C2 has spread farther.

The TNM System is more specific about the location of the cancer. It has just recently been updated, so we refer to it as the "new" TNM System. In this system:

▶ **T** stands for "tumor." When a tumor is staged, the pathologist's report will include a capital T with a number between 1 and 4, and a lowercase letter (a, b, or c) next to it. The greater the number and letter, the farther the cancer has spread. For example, a T2b cancer is confined to the prostate but covers more area than a T2a cancer. A T3b cancer has spread a little beyond the prostate, while a T4 cancer has spread far beyond the prostate. If a cancer other than prostate cancer is detected, then the report may include a capital T with a zero (T0).

TABLE I-3.—The ABCD and New TNM Clinical Staging Systems for Localized Prostate Cancer

ABCD	TNM	What Do the Results Mean?
—	TX	The cancer cannot be staged at this time.
—	T0	There is no evidence of a cancer.
A	T1	A cancer that cannot be felt with a DRE or picked up by an imaging machine (X-ray, CT scan, MRI, etc.) or is found by PSA or another procedure, such as a TURP for BPH. This is "localized or confined prostate cancer."
A1	T1a	A cancer that is found during a procedure such as a TURP (not found by a biopsy). The cancer takes up less than 5% of prostate tissue removed in the procedure.
A2	T1b	A cancer that is found during a procedure such as a TURP. The cancer takes up more than 5% of the prostate tissue removed in the procedure.
B0	T1c	A cancer that cannot be felt with a DRE but it is detected by a biopsy in one or both sides of the prostate, because of an initial high PSA level.
B1 or B2	T2	The cancer is only confined or within the prostate, and/or it has invaded the apex of the prostate (where the urethra leaves the prostate), or it has gone into but not beyond the prostate capsule. This is still called a "localized or confined prostate cancer."
B1	T2a	A cancer that occupies only one side (lobe) of the prostate.
B2	T2b	A cancer that occupies both sides (lobes) of the prostate.

NOTE: There is no longer a T2c cancer with the newer system.

TABLE I-4.—The ABCD and New TNM Clinical Staging Systems for Advanced Prostate Cancer

ABCD	TNM	What Do the Results Mean?
C1–C2	T3	The cancer goes through the prostate capsule. This is also called "locally advanced prostate disease."
C1	T3a	A cancer on one or both sides of the prostate that is now growing on the outside and going beyond the prostate. this is also called "unilateral (one side) or bilateral (both sides) extracapsular extension."
C2	T3b	A cancer that has invaded one or both seminal vesicles.

Note: There is no longer a T3c cancer with the newer system.

ABCD	TNM	What Do the Results Mean?
C2	T4	A cancer that has spread to or invaded other nearby structures other than the seminal vesicle(s) such as the: bladder neck, external sphincter, rectum, nearby muscles (also called "levator muscles") and/or the pelvic wall. This is also called a "locally or regionally advanced prostate cancer."

Note: There is no longer a T4a or T4b prostate cancer with the newer system.

ABCD	TNM	What Do the Results Mean?
—	NX	The lymph nodes cannot be staged at this time.
—	N0	No lymph nodes near the prostate have cancer (or metastasis). These are also called "regional lymph nodes."
D1	N1	Cancer in a regional node or nodes near the prostate. This is also called a "regionally advanced prostate cancer."

Note: There is no longer a N2 or N3 prostate cancer or an N+ cancer with the newer system.

Note: The regional lymph nodes are in the pelvic area and there are 5 sets of them called: Pelvic, Hypogastric, Obturator, Iliac, and Sacral.

		TABLE I-4.—Continued
ABCD	**TNM**	**What Do the Results Mean?**
—	MX	Metastasis or cancer spread far beyond the prostate (also called "distant metastasis") cannot be staged at this time.
—	MO	There is no metastasis or cancer spread far beyond the prostate (also called "no distant metastasis").
D2	M1	Cancer has metastasized or spread far beyond the prostate (also called "distant metastasis"). This is also called and "Advanced Prostate Cancer."
D2	M1a	Cancer has metastasized or spread to a node or nodes far beyond the prostate (also called "nonregional lymph node or nodes").
D2	M1b	Cancer has metastasized or spread to the bone or bones.
D2	M1c	Cancer has metastasized or spread to another site or sites in the body far beyond the prostate (such as the liver, lungs, and bones). This is the most advanced category or stage of prostate cancer.

Note: The newer staging system has added an M1b and M1c category and has eliminated the M+ category.

Note: The nonregional lymph nodes are far from the prostate and there are 8 sets of them called: Aortic (also called "para-aortic lumbar"); Common iliac; Inguinal; Superficial inguinal (also called "femoral"); Supraclavicular; Cervical; Scalene; and Retroperitoneal.

Note: M or Metastasis, or cancer spread far beyond the prostate commonly goes to the bone or bones. In addition, during metastasis, the cancer can commonly go to nonregional or distant lymph nodes. Prostate cancer to the lung is uncommon with metastasis but when it occurs it usually is because it has gone along the distant lymph nodes to eventually reach the lung. Liver metastasis or cancer that has spread to the liver is very uncommon and it usually occurs late in the course of this disease.

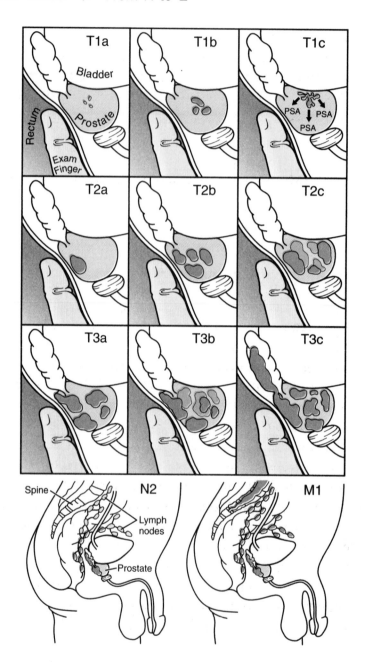

FIGURE I-7.—The progression of prostate cancer, from the earliest stages to the most advanced, along with the corresponding TNM and ABCD stages. Keep in mind that the T2c and T3c examples shown above are no longer a part of the newer staging system.

► **N** stands for "nodes." If the lymph nodes contain cancer, the staging report will include a capital N (for nodes) with a plus sign next to it: "N+," as well as a T. If the lymph nodes do not contain cancer, the report will include a capital N with a zero (N0). An "x"(Nx) is used if the status of the lymph nodes is not known.

► **M** stands for "metastasis." If the cancer has spread far beyond the prostate—to the bones, for example—then the staging report will include a capital M. If the cancer has not spread far beyond the prostate, the report may include a capital M with a zero (M0). An "x"(Mx) is used if it is unknown whether or not someone has metastatic disease.

► Clinical Staging and Pathological Staging

The ABCD and TNM systems are "clinical staging" methods for a cancer based on clinical information, such as a DRE, a PSA test, ultrasound tests, etc. Clinical staging is really only an estimate of how far a cancer has spread, and it is never 100% accurate.

As a result, the stage of cancer can be underestimated or overestimated in clinical staging. For example, doctors may believe that a cancer is T3 based on the clinical information, but in reality it may turn out to be a T2 or relatively confined prostate cancer. In that case, the cancer would have been overestimated or "overstaged." On the other hand, someone may have been identified as having a clinical stage of T2, but actually turn out to have a T3. Here, the cancer has been "understaged." The problem is that such inaccuracies can lead to the use of ineffective treatment, or to lost treatment opportunities. As with the grading of cancers, about 25% of people have their cancers overstaged, and another 25% or so have them understaged. In the hands of an experienced physician, the chance of being accurately staged through clinical methods is very good.

The most accurate way to determine how far a cancer has spread is through pathological staging—that is, by actually looking at samples of all the tissue in question. But there's a catch: The only patients who are candidates for pathological staging are those who have had a radical prostatectomy, which provides the pathologist with the tissue to examine.

There is a system created specifically for pathological staging. Known as "pT," this system describes the spread of cancer to areas around the prostate. It does not encompass areas far beyond the prostate, because there are other techniques, such as imaging and biopsies that are used to identify cancer in the bones, lungs, liver, etc.

▶ Surgical Margins

When a surgeon cuts around the prostate during a radical prostatectomy, the prostate and the areas removed with it are sent to a pathologist for examination. The pathologist looks at the outer edges of the sample—the margins—to see if cancer is present. If it is, there is a greater chance that it has spread beyond the area removed during surgery. If those margins do not contain cancer, there is a greater possibility that the cancer is

TABLE I-5.—The Pathologic Staging System. Also known as pT.*	
Pathologic Stage	**What Does that Really mean?**
pT2	This is a localized or prostate (organ) confined cancer.
pT2a	This is a prostate cancer that is localized or confined to only one side of the prostate. It is also called a "unilateral" prostate cancer.
pT2b	This is a prostate cancer that is localized or confined to both sides of the prostate. It is also called a "bilateral" prostate cancer.
pT3	This is a prostate cancer that has spread just beyond the prostate. It is also called "extraprostatic extension."
pT3a	This is a prostate cancer that has barely spread beyond the prostate. It is also called "extraprostatic extension."
pT3b	This is a prostate cancer that has spread to the seminal vesicle(s), which are located near the prostate.
pT4	This is a prostate cancer that has spread to the bladder and/or rectum.

Note: There is no pathologic T1 category and there is no category beyond T4. For example, there is no pN (for lymph nodes) and there is no pM (for metastatic spread).

* The small "p" means "pathologic" while the capital "T" means "Tumor."

EXAMPLE PATHOLOGICAL REPORT

Tissue Evaluation

Prostate size _____ cm x _____ cm x _____ cm

Prostate weight _____ g

Seminal vesicles size _____ cm x _____ cm x _____ cm

Seminal vesicles weight _____ g

Unilateral cancer? _____   Bilateral cancer? _____

Pelvic lymphadenectomy tissue submitted?_____

Diagnosis

Radical prostatectomy?_____   Retropubic?_____   Perineal?_____

Adenocarcinoma

   Gleason Grade _____ + _____ = _____

   Gleason Grade _____ pattern: _____ %

   Gleason Grade _____ pattern: _____ %

   Size _____ cc

Location: Unilateral? _____   Bilateral? _____

Peripheral Zone? _____   and/or Central Zone? _____

                                and/or Transition Zone? _____

Surgical or resection margins   Positive? _____   Negative? _____

Capsule involvement?   Within capsule? _____   Beyond capsule? _____

                              Unifocal? _____   Multifocal? _____

Perineural invasion? _____

Premalignant change? _____   High-grade PIN? _____

Pelvic lymph nodes? _____   Cancer? _____

How many nodes are positive? _____

Prostate Apex? _____   Positive? _____   Negative? _____

Bladder base? _____   Positive? _____   Negative? _____

Vascular/lymphatic involvement?

                        Yes? _____ / extensive? _____   No? _____

TNM stage?   Tumor? _____   Nodes? _____   Metastasis? _____

Other observations: BPH? _____   Prostatitis? _____

Optional

Cores: Number of cores taken? _____

         Number positive? _____

           Total length of cancer in any core? _____

           Percent of cancer in each core? _____

DNA content: Diploid? ____   Aneuploid? ____   Tetraploid? ____

Note: Some of this information can come from the biopsy. Obviously these reports differ somewhat from hospital to hospital. However, this is some of the standard information it should contain.

A SECOND TYPE OF PATHOLOGICAL REPORT

Mapping Report

Location	Diagnosis	Core Length (mm)	Tumor Length (mm)	Percent Tumor	Tumor Position from Inked Margin
Left Apex (Core 1/1)	4 + 3 = 7	10	9.0	90	Not Inked
Left Seminal Vesicle (Core 1/2)	4 + 3 = 7	6	6.0	100	Not Inked
Left Seminal Vesicle (Core 2/2)	4 + 3 = 7	8	1.0	12	Not Inked
Left Mid (Core 1/1)	4 + 3 = 7	12	4.0	33	Not Inked
Right Base (Core 1/1)	4 + 3 = 7	15	5.0	33	Not Inked
Right Mid (Core 1/1)	4 + 3 = 7	12	2.0	16	Not Inked

Note: In this example, the patient has a Gleason score of 4 + 3 = 7, with locally advanced disease to one seminal vesicle.

confined to the prostate. Therefore, the pathologist may report that the prostate is margin positive (+), meaning that some cancer was found in the margins, or that the prostate is margin negative (-), which means no cancer was found in the margins.

Many men who have had a biopsy or surgery to remove the prostate keep a copy of their pathology report for their records. This report gives a clear idea of how far the cancer has spread and just how aggressive it is.

What is the Difference between Localized, Locally-Advanced, Regionally-Advanced, and Advanced or Metastatic Prostate Cancer?

The various stages of cancer are determined by if, and how far the cancer has spread outside of the prostate.

▶ **Localized Cancer:** Cancer that has not grown beyond the prostate. It is also known as stage T1 or T2 in the TNM system, or stage A or B in the ABCD system.

▶ **Locally-Advanced Prostate Cancer:** Cancer that has grown just beyond the prostate and/or spread to neighboring tissues, such as the seminal vesicles (stage T3 or C). This also includes cases where the cancer has spread to nearby organs, such as the rectum or bladder (T4 or C). Basically, the term "locally-advanced cancer" covers all those cancers that are stage T3 or stage T4, or C.

▶ **Regionally-Advanced Cancer:** Cancer that has spread to the lymph nodes. This is also known as N1 or D1 prostate cancer.

▶ **Advanced or Metastatic Cancer:** Cancer that has spread far beyond the prostate or local lymph nodes to lymph nodes farther from the prostate, or to bones and/or other organs (M1 or D2). However, advanced prostate cancer can also be divided into those cancers that are androgen-dependent (also known as "hormone-insensitive," hormone-refractory," or AIPC, which stands for Androgen-Independent Prostate Cancer).

▶ **Recurrence** applies to those cases in which treatment has not been effective. In other words, if after treatment the cancer is not cured or the PSA begins to increase. This is not a true cancer stage, but it is useful because it describes a specific situation. Recurring cancer can still be confined to the prostate, or it may have spread to the area around the prostate.

Regardless of what advanced prostate cancer is called, there are many options that must be carefully examined and discussed with the doctor before choosing the right treatment.

MAKING THE MOST OF DOCTOR VISITS

J

The time spent with the doctor is critically important, but it is also limited. The following rules will help someone make decisions.

▶ **RULE I:** BE PREPARED

▶ **RULE II:** BRING SUPPORT

▶ **RULE III:** ASK QUESTIONS

▶ **RULE IV:** TAKE NOTES

▶ **RULE V:** HAVE REALISTIC EXPECTATIONS

Rule I: Be Prepared

Often, doctors spend a lot of time explaining the basics, which can take valuable time. The more someone learns before an office visit, the more time there will be to ask the doctor important questions.

Before an appointment with the doctor, consider making preparations such as:

Make a written list of questions.

▶ Update knowledge of tests and treatments.

▶ Review medical records. Consider keeping a health journal, and create a summary of PSA results (along with treatments) over the past year or two.

▶ Ask the doctor what should be brought to the next appointment. For example, are copies of medical records or test results needed?

▶ Review medical insurance coverage. For example, does it pay for experimental treatments? What sort of deductible is there?

▶ Do not be afraid to tape record the appointment (as long as you have your doctor's permission).

Rule II: Bring Support

It is a good idea to bring someone along to a doctor's appointment. The emotional and mental assistance this provides is invaluable. Also, for example, it is not uncommon for a spouse or partner to remember important details and questions during a visit. They can also be affected mentally and physically. Doctors and therapists can greatly assist a couple during this difficult time.

Rule III: Ask Questions

Bring a written list of questions to a doctor's appointment. It is important to focus on the most important questions, because surveys have shown that only about 25% of the questions brought in by patients are actually answered. So, write down the top five or ten. For example, an important question might be, "What is the success rate with this treatment?" And a less important question might be, "How soon after the treatment can golf be played again?"

Never be afraid to tell or ask the doctor anything. Questions that seem embarrassing are probably routine for the doctor. If the doctor does not want to provide certain information, or seems to discourage questions, it might be time to find another doctor. Communication and mutual respect are important components of a successful doctor-patient relationship.

Rule IV: Take Notes

Total recall of what occurred during an office visit is virtually impossible. Always bring a paper and a pen to a doctor's appointment as there will usually be a lot to remember. Another option is to tape record the session for future reference.

Rule V: Have Realistic Expectations

Evaluate all the information before making a decision on anything, carefully weighing the pros and cons of each course of action. The opinions of the doctors, spouse or partner, support group members, books, and other sources are all parts of the total picture and important considerations in any decision. There is no single definitive treatment for prostate cancer and treatment possibilities are continuing to evolve and grow. So, do not take one person's advice or experience as the final word. Instead, consider getting opinions:

- From several doctors.
- From individuals who have been in a similar situation.
- From spouses or partners who have watched their mate go through the treatment.
- From books, articles, and the Internet.

Every prostate cancer treatment has its good points and bad points. Insist on knowing all the pros and cons of treatments, and inquire about:

- Financial cost.
- Potential side effects. That means not just general or overall side effects, but specifically those that can be expected from each procedure. Ask what percentage of the doctor's patients experience side effects and how long those side effects last. Also,

ask the doctor to define the words being used. For example, if the a side effect is impotence, does that mean temporary or permanent impotence? Complete or partial loss of erectile function? Words mean different things to different doctors.

▶ How is the side effect normally treated? Would a medication correct it? Does it usually go away with time? Would surgery be needed to correct it?

▶ What is the doctor's success rate with this treatment? How is success measured? By PSA level? By other lab values? By months or years of living longer?

▶ If it is a new test, how accurate is it? What percentage of participants gets false positives or false negatives? What conditions make it more likely to get a false reading? Is this the best time to have this test done?

▶ Does it decrease pain or improve mobility? Does it increase life expectancy? Does the treatment affect or interact with other existing medical conditions? For example, if someone has early signs of osteoporosis, hormonal therapy could make the osteoporosis worse. If there is a potential problem, are there ways to minimize the risk?

▶ Can alternative treatments affect treatment? Can they be used in combination with conventional treatment?

▶ Is the treatment FDA-approved or is it experimental? If it is experimental, why hasn't it been approved by the FDA?

Question the doctor closely if the treatment or test recommended is the only option. At nearly every stage of prostate cancer, there are many options to consider. Make sure the doctor gives a thorough, objective explanation of them all. These five rules will help someone get the most out of an appointment with a doctor and at the same time will serve to empower them with the most knowledge about their cancer.

The key to a good doctor visit can also be found in the word

P–R–O–S–T–A–T–E

The following memory device may be helpful:

Preparation. Read a number of articles or books about prostate cancer before seeing a doctor. Review medical insurance. Does it cover the cost of any experimental treatments? Does it pay for all medications and tests? If not, how much does the insurance cover? Unfortunately for most, medical costs are an important equation in the treatment decision-making process.

Knowledge is power when it comes to prostate cancer, so be well prepared for an office visit.

Realistic Expectations. When it comes to prostate cancer, if a treatment sounds too good to be true, then it definitely is. Always find out the disadvantages—what the "catch" is—for a specific treatment before making any decision. Insist the doctor emphasize the pros and cons of a particular treatment.

Opinions. Seek as many opinions as possible. Do not take one person's advice as absolute, no matter who it is. Listen to as many viewpoints as possible before making an informed decision.

Also get information from a support group or attend a meeting. Many times the meetings will have guest speakers who provide free, up-to-date medical information. Talk to the group members or at least a few men who have gone through a similar experience. If the doctor provides a list of men to talk to that is fine, but also seek out men not on the list. Feel free to take advantage of such resources to learn as much as possible about the disease and its treatment.

Spousal or Partner Support. A mate, family member or friend should be brought to the doctor's appointment. Having someone there helps not only provides emotional support but they may bring up additional questions or remember something else. Also, talk to the doctor about how this process may affect the support person and what that person can do to help make the situation better. Encourage the support person to talk to others who have been in a similar situation to gain insight on how to best cope with caring for a man with prostate cancer.

Take Notes. Bring a pad of paper and a pen to the appointment. Bringing a tape recorder is a good idea, too.

Ask. Bring a written list of questions. A list greatly increases the chances of getting wanted information.

Talk. Feel free to tell the doctor anything or to ask any type of question, including matters such as sexual functioning and incontinence. These topics are routine for the doctor.

Evaluate. After collecting information, take time to evaluate it. Discuss this information with someone. Make an informed treatment decision.

NOTES

Section

3

Treatment of Localized Prostate Cancer

HOW DOCTORS EVALUATE
THE EFFECTIVENESS
OF VARIOUS
TREATMENTS

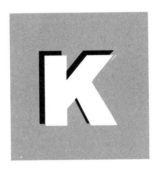

Doctors have several ways of gauging the success of a particular prostate cancer treatment. These are often called "end points" because they describe the end outcome of treatment. These end points usually look at treatment in one of two ways:

1. The percentage of men receiving the procedure who can expect a successful outcome.

2. The percentage of men receiving the procedure who can expect an outcome that is not successful.

The doctor that will perform a procedure can provide specific end points—that is, how successful they have been with the procedure. These end points can be compared with the average end points from the medical literature.

However, there are a couple of important things to bear in mind. For one, many of the procedures used to treat prostate cancer are fairly new, so they may not have established much of a long-term record. Also, procedures are evolving all the time, so past results may not provide a completely accurate view of the future.

Above all, remember that these end points are statistics that tend to describe the "average" person. These statistics are often based on a wide variety of cases and on predictions and probabilities, and they rely on studies that cover varying lengths of time. Statistics can be helpful in making decisions about treatment, but they can never predict precisely what will happen to a specific individual.

There are many end points used by doctors today.

Some of the more common ones are:

▶ **Overall Survival Rates.** This indicates how long individuals usually live after a given treatment, and it includes any cause of death. For example, if someone lives for 20 years after prostate cancer surgery and dies of heart disease or is hit by a car, he is counted. Therefore, this is not a very precise assessment of the success of a procedure.

▶ **Cancer-Specific Survival Rates ~ (also called) Cancer Survival:** This looks at the people who die of cancer after being treated for it. For example, if the cancer-specific survival rate for a procedure is 50% at 10 years, it means that the average man who receives this procedure can expect to survive at least 10 years before he dies from prostate cancer. This is a more precise way to describe the effectiveness of a procedure than the overall survival rate.

▶ **Freedom from Metastasis, or Metastatic-Free Disease:** This looks at how long the average man can expect to be free from advanced disease after a procedure. For example, if 95% of the men receiving this procedure have freedom from metastasis for 15 years, this indicates that it is very effective. It also means that 5% of the men who have this procedure can expect to experience metastasis within 15 years.

▶ **Freedom from Local Recurrence:** This looks at the length of time after a procedure that someone can expect to be free of localized cancer. For example, 80% of the individuals studied had freedom from local recurrence after 10 years, which is pretty good. The use of this measurement suggests that the procedure was performed with the hope of eliminating all of the cancer.

▶ **Freedom from any Recurrence:** This is the percentage of individuals who did not have a recurrence of cancer after a certain period of time, or the length of time after a procedure that it typically takes for signs of recurring cancer to appear.

▶ **Freedom from Biochemical or PSA Recurrence ~ (also called)**

Biochemical Relapse-Free Survival, Detectable PSA, or Subclinical Progression: The PSA level should be zero after surgery or close to zero after a procedure such as radiation, so this assesses how long it takes for PSA levels to become detectable again (the rise of PSA levels suggests that the cancer has returned). This is probably the most accurate way to gauge the success of prostate cancer treatments, since a rising PSA will often show up long before other clinical signs, such as a positive DRE, bone scan, or serum acid phosphatase levels—as long as three to six years before, in some cases.

It is important to note that the meaning of "freedom from PSA recurrence" can vary depending on the individual doctor or the procedure in question. For example, after a radical prostatectomy there should be an undetectable PSA or one that is nearly zero (some say less than or equal to 0.2). After a radiation, or treatment, on the other hand, the PSA level used to determine freedom from PSA recurrence varies from doctor to doctor.

▶ **Progression-Free Survival:** This looks at the percentage of people who can expect to have their cancer remain at the same stage—that is, not advance any further—after a procedure.

▶ **Partial and Complete Disease Regression:** Regression literally means "going back," so this is the percentage of individuals who can expect to have their cancer regress somewhat or completely after the procedure or treatment. It is generally used in regard to treatment with hormones or chemotherapy. Reports might show that five years after treatment, 75% of the men with cancer in the nodes had partial or complete disappearance of that cancer, which is a pretty good record. It is important to keep in mind that there is a difference between partial and complete regression. Partial regression means that the cancer is still in a certain location in the body, but there is less of it than there was prior to the procedure. Complete regression means that the cancer is no longer at that site after the procedure.

WATCHFUL WAITING OR EXPECTANT MANAGEMENT

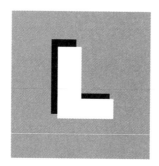

WATCHFUL WAITING IS JUST THAT—
WATCHING AND WAITING . . .
THIS APPROACH HAS MANY NAMES

- ▶ CONSERVATIVE THERAPY
- ▶ DELAYED THERAPY
- ▶ EXPECTANT MANAGEMENT
- ▶ NO THERAPY
- ▶ SURVEILLANCE
- ▶ WITHOUT SPECIFIC THERAPY

Watchful waiting does not mean that nothing is done. It means that even though someone has decided not to have treatment, the prostate cancer is still being regularly monitored through PSA testing, DRE, and/or TRUS. The word "regular" means an examination at least every six months. The doctor may also want to do a biopsy once a year or more to get a better idea of the cancer's aggressiveness. It also means that as soon as any change is detected, more active treatment can begin.

The best candidates for watchful waiting are:

▶ Men whose life expectancy is no more than 10 years due to age (such as those over 75), or other medical illnesses.

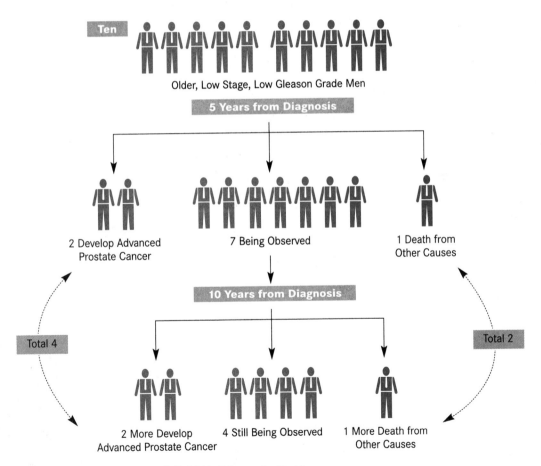

Ten

Older, Low Stage, Low Gleason Grade Men

5 Years from Diagnosis

2 Develop Advanced Prostate Cancer

7 Being Observed

1 Death from Other Causes

10 Years from Diagnosis

Total 4

Total 2

2 More Develop Advanced Prostate Cancer

4 Still Being Observed

1 More Death from Other Causes

FIGURE L-1.—Watchful Waiting statistics.

▶   Men over the age of 70 with a well-differentiated (Gleason score of 2– 4), and very small cancer.

▶   Men whose cancer is confined to the prostate and who want to take time to decide on the type of treatment.

▶   Men who have advanced prostate cancer (cancer that has spread beyond the prostate gland) and have not experienced symptoms.

The advantages of watchful waiting:

▶   Side effects or complications associated with any of the treatments for prostate cancer are avoided.

▶   It is the least expensive option in the short term. The only costs associated with this management approach involve regular PSA testing, DRE, and occasional prostate biopsies, which total about $1,200 a year. However, if the prostate cancer spreads, then the long-term costs of treatment could easily outweigh the short-term savings.

▶   It permits time for calm and rational treatment decisions. Prostate cancer can be a very slow-growing malignancy. When it is confined to the prostate, it can take several years for it to double in size. Therefore, under certain circumstances, there are benefits to watchful waiting.

The disadvantage of watchful waiting:

▶   It allows the cancer to continue to grow. And even for cancers that are not aggressive or large, it can still be a risk because any cancer can potentially change its characteristics at any time. A cancer that has a Gleason score of 4 today could remain at 4 or develop into a 5 or 7 (less likely but possible).

Studies indicate that watchful waiting is an adequate treatment option for older men with low-grade cancers (Gleason score 2–4). However, older men with moderate (Gleason score 5–7) or high-grade cancer (Gleason score 8–10) should consider receiving some kind of treatment.

Watchful waiting is used in relatively few patients with locally-advanced cancer. However, it is an option for older patients with a life expectancy of less than 10 years and low to moderate Gleason scores.

Studies have shown that watchful waiting works in terms of "Cancer-Specific Survival":

▶ Among men with a low total Gleason score (2–4), 2% die of cancer within 5 years, and 10% within 10 years.

▶ Among men with a moderate total Gleason score (5–7), 3% die of cancer after 5 years, and 13% after 10 years.

▶ Among men with high total Gleason score (8–10), 33% die of cancer after 5 years and 66% will die after 10 years.

Basically, the lower the Gleason score, the more likely it is that watchful waiting will succeed.

In terms of "Metastasis-Free Survival" and watchful waiting, studies have shown the following results:

▶ Among men with low-grade cancer, only 7% have metastasis after 5 years, and 19% within 10 years.

▶ Among men with moderate-grade cancer, 16% have metastasis within 5 years, and 42% within 10 years.

▶ Among men with high-grade cancer, 49% have metastasis after 5 years, and 74% with 10 years.

SURGERY

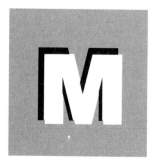

Until quite recently, up to 90% of men who underwent complete surgical removal of the prostate, or radical prostatectomy, were left without sexual function and up to 20% became incontinent. The majority also experienced significant blood loss during surgery, requiring several transfusions.

In the past decade, however, a more refined approach to prostate-removal surgery has become widespread. This "nerve-sparing" or "anatomical" approach, developed in the early 1980s by Patrick Walsh, M.D., of Johns Hopkins University, involves using long, thin surgical instruments to cut free and protect the nerves and valves surrounding the prostate that control sexual function and urination.

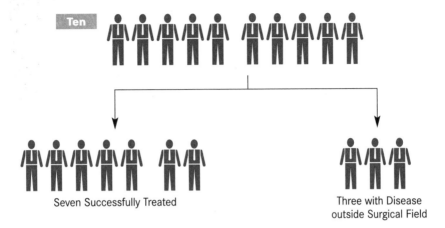

FIGURE M-1.—Surgery statistics.

	After 5 Years	After 10 Years	After 15 Years
TABLE M–1.—The Effectiveness of Radical Prostatectomy for Localized Prostate Cancer (T2)			
Statistics	**After 5 Years**	**After 10 Years**	**After 15 Years**
Percentage of men still alive (overall survival)	69–95%	44–88%	22–75%
Percentage of men who have not died of prostate cancer (disease-specific or cause-specific survival)	90–97%	88–93%	55–93%
Percentage of men whose cancer has progressed (metastasis)	8–18%	18%	30%

Note:
Cancer characteristics of these patients: 23% had well-differentiated, 57% had moderately differentiated, and 20% had poorly differentiated cancers.

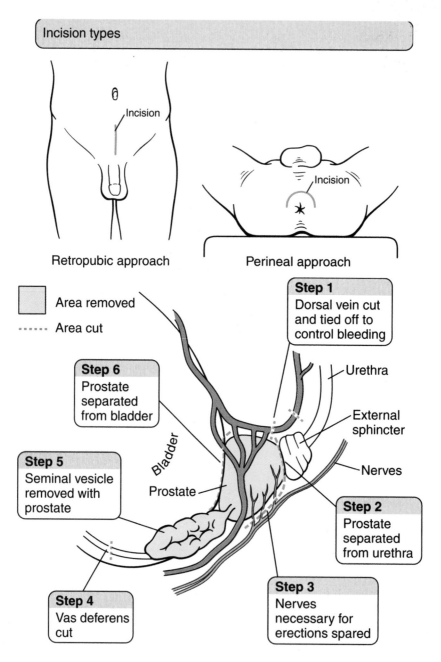

FIGURE M-2a.—The incisions used in the two types of radical prostatectomy, the order in which the surgeon carries out the procedure,
and the final reconstuction process in the surgery, which takes about
three hours.

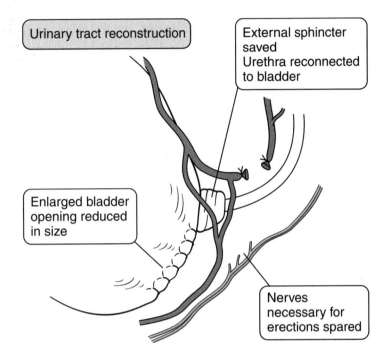

Urinary tract reconstruction

External sphincter saved
Urethra reconnected to bladder

Enlarged bladder opening reduced in size

Nerves necessary for erections spared

FIGURE M-2b.—Radical prostatectomy *(continued)*.

The Special Case of a Rising PSA after a Radical Prostatectomy

Unfortunately, radical prostatectomy is not always successful in curing cancer. This may be due to microscopic disease that was not removed at the time of surgery. The cancer then begins once more to grow as a local recurrence. If there is no evidence of distant metastases (negative bone scan, negative CT scan), radiation should be considered as a curative salvage treatment. Studies have demonstrated that radiation works better the lower the PSA (<1–2).

The ability to have an erection is controlled by nerve bundles located on each side of the prostate. Whether one or both of these nerve bundles can be spared during surgery depends on the extent and location of the cancer. If the cancer is located centrally, away from the outer surface of the gland, then both nerve bundles can be spared. If the cancer is on one side, then only one nerve bundle needs to be removed. If both sides of the prostate are cancerous, then both nerve bundles must go. The nerves on both sides are also traditionally removed in men who already suffer from impotence, or the inability to achieve an erection, at the time of surgery. Since their nerve bundles are no longer needed, it is not necessary to save them.

A man can still have an erection if only one nerve bundle is removed. If both are removed, a man can still have a normal sex drive, sensation, and orgasm, but cannot have a normal erection. However, even if both sets of nerves have been removed, with the help of certain devices and medications, a man can achieve an erection as good as before surgery.

It is important to note that after the prostate is removed, ejaculations will be "dry," which means very little fluid will come out. This is because the prostate and the seminal vesicles, which are removed during surgery, make most of the seminal fluid, which carries sperm from the testicles. Therefore, if a man wants to father a child, a needle aspiration of sperm from the testicles can be done. The sperm is then used for in-vitro fertilization. This technique has about a 30% success rate.

There are three types of Nerve-Sparing or Anatomical Radical Prostatectomy:

Radical Retropubic Prostatectomy. This is the most common type of prostate-removal surgery, accounting for 85% of all such operations. In this procedure, a vertical incision is made about an inch above the penis (in front of the pubic bone) up to the navel, or belly button. At the beginning of the operation, the pelvic lymph nodes can be removed through this incision and examined to determine whether or not the cancer has spread beyond the prostate. If the lymph nodes are clear, the operation continues. If they are cancerous, the operation is discontinued and other treatment methods are explored.

Radical Perineal Prostatectomy. This is an operation in which a semicircular incision is made between the scrotum (the pouch that holds the testicles) and the anus. If the pelvic lymph nodes need to be examined, a separate incision must be made in the lower abdomen. In general, there is less bleeding with this type of prostatectomy and heavier men fare better with this approach. Also, there is no visible scar in the abdominal area. However, it is more difficult to save the nerve bundles—and thus erectile function—with this type of surgery.

Radical Laparoscopic Prostatectomy. Talk with your doctor about the advantages and disadvantages of this procedure.

Regardless of which style of radical prostatectomy is chosen, the outcome and side effects depend largely on who is doing the surgery. That is why it is important to select a surgeon who has been properly trained and performs this surgery regularly. The earlier a cancer is detected and the less aggressive it is, the better chance there is for a cure. Tables (pages 124–127) and nomograms (page 129) have been developed that can help predict if an operation will be successful in removing all of the cancer based on preoperative PSA, Gleason Score, and pathologic stage.

If after surgery the PSA level increases or the cancer returns, then radiation therapy is still a treatment option.

The best candidates for Radical Prostatectomy are:

▶ Men who are expected to live at least 10 more years (usually those under age 70).
▶ Men whose cancer is confined to prostate gland.

Those who generally do not qualify for Radical Prostatectomy are:

▶ Men with a life expectancy of less than 10 years.
▶ Men who suffer from other serious medical conditions, such as congestive heart failure.
▶ Men whose cancer has spread beyond the prostate.

The advantages of Radical Prostatectomy:

▶ It can potentially cure prostate cancer.
▶ It allows the cancer to be accurately staged through pathological examination of the tumor specimen.
▶ The PSA test can be used as an accurate predictor of whether the cancer has been completely removed or if it has returned.
▶ If surgery fails then radiation therapy is still an option (but not vice versa).

TABLE M-2.—Clinical Stage T1c (nonpalpable, PSA elevated)

PSA Range (ng/mL)	Pathologic Stage	Gleason Score				
		2–4	5–6	3 + 4 = 7	4 + 3 = 7	8–10
0–2.5	Organ confined	95 (89–99)	90 (88–93)	79 (74–85)	71 (62–79)	66 (54–76)
	Extraprostatic extension	5 (1–11)	9 (7–12)	17 (13–23)	25 (18–34)	28 (20–38)
	Seminal vesicle (+)	—	0 (0–1)	2 (1–5)	2 (1–5)	4 (1–10)
	Lymph node (+)	—	—	1 (0–2)	1 (0–4)	1 (0–4)
2.6–4.0	Organ confined	92 (82–98)	84 (81–86)	68 (62–74)	58 (48–67)	52 (41–63)
	Extraprostatic extension	8 (2–18)	15 (13–18)	27 (22–33)	37 (29–46)	40 (31–50)
	Seminal vesicle (+)	—	1 (0–1)	4 (2–7)	4 (1–7)	6 (3–12)
	Lymph node (+)	—	—	1 (0–2)	1 (0–3)	1 (0–4)
4.1–6.0	Organ confined	90 (78–98)	80 (78–83)	63 (58–68)	52 (43–60)	46 (36–56)
	Extraprostatic extension	10 (2–22)	19 (16–21)	32 (27–36)	42 (35–50)	45 (36–54)
	Seminal vesicle (+)	—	1 (0–1)	3 (2–5)	3 (1–6)	5 (3–9)
	Lymph node (+)	—	0 (0–1)	2 (1–3)	3 (1–5)	3 (1–6)
6.1–10.0	Organ confined	87 (73–97)	75 (72–77)	54 (49–59)	43 (35–51)	37 (28–46)
	Extraprostatic extension	13 (3–27)	23 (21–25)	36 (32–40)	47 (40–54)	48 (39–57)
	Seminal vesicle (+)	—	2 (2–3)	8 (6–11)	8 (4–12)	13 (8–19)
	Lymph node (+)	—	0 (0–1)	2 (1–3)	2 (1–4)	3 (1–5)
>10.0	Organ confined	80 (61–95)	62 (58–64)	37 (32–42)	27 (21–34)	22 (16–30)
	Extraprostatic extension	20 (5–39)	33 (30–36)	43 (38–48)	51 (44–59)	50 (42–59)
	Seminal vesicle (+)	—	4 (3–5)	12 (9–17)	11 (6–17)	17 (10–25)
	Lymph node (+)	—	2 (1–3)	8 (5–11)	10 (5–17)	11 (5–18)

TABLE M-3.—Clinical Stage T2a (palpable < of one lobe)

PSA Range (ng/mL)	Pathologic Stage	Gleason Score				
		2-4	5-6	3 + 4 = 7	4 + 3 = 7	8-10
0-2.5	Organ confined	91 (79-98)	81 (77-85)	64 (56-71)	53 (43-63)	47 (35-59)
	Extraprostatic extension	9 (2-21)	17 (13-21)	29 (23-36)	40 (30-49)	42 (32-53)
	Seminal vesicle (+)	—	1 (0-2)	5 (1-9)	4 (1-9)	7 (2-16)
	Lymph node (+)	—	0 (0-1)	2 (0-5)	3 (0-8)	3 (0-9)
2.6-4.0	Organ confined	85 (69-96)	71 (66-75)	50 (43-57)	39 (30-48)	33 (24-44)
	Extraprostatic extension	15 (4-31)	27 (23-31)	41 (35-48)	52 (43-61)	53 (44-63)
	Seminal vesicle (+)	—	2 (1-3)	7 (3-12)	6 (2-12)	10 (4-18)
	Lymph node (+)	—	0 (0-1)	2 (0-4)	2 (0-6)	3 (0-8)
4.1-6.0	Organ confined	81 (63-95)	66 (62-70)	44 (39-50)	33 (25-41)	28 (20-37)
	Extraprostatic extension	19 (5-37)	32 (28-36)	46 (40-52)	56 (48-64)	58 (49-66)
	Seminal vesicle (+)	—	1 (1-2)	5 (3-8)	5 (2-8)	8 (4-13)
	Lymph node (+)	—	1 (0-2)	4 (2-7)	6 (3-11)	6 (2-12)
6.1-10.0	Organ confined	76 (56-94)	58 (54-61)	35 (30-40)	25 (19-32)	21 (15-28)
	Extraprostatic extension	24 (6-44)	37 (34-41)	49 (43-54)	58 (51-66)	57 (48-65)
	Seminal vesicle (+)	—	4 (3-5)	13 (9-18)	11 (6-17)	17 (11-26)
	Lymph node (+)	—	1 (0-2)	3 (2-6)	5 (2-8)	5 (2-10)
>10.0	Organ confined	65 (43-89)	42 (38-46)	20 (17-24)	14 (10-18)	11 (7-15)
	Extraprostatic extension	35 (11-57)	47 (43-52)	49 (43-55)	55 (46-64)	52 (41-62)
	Seminal vesicle (+)	—	6 (4-8)	16 (11-022)	13 (7-30)	19 (12-29)
	Lymph node (+)	—	4 (3-7)	14 (9-21)	18 (10-27)	17 (9-29)

TABLE M-4.—Clinical Stage T2b (palpable > of one lobe, not on both lobes)

PSA Range (ng/mL)	Pathologic Stage	Gleason Score				
		2–4	5–6	3 + 4 = 7	4 + 3 = 7	8–10
0–2.5	Organ confined	88 (73–97)	75 (69–81)	54 (46–63)	43 (33–54)	37 (26–49)
	Extraprostatic extension	12 (3–27)	22 (17280)	35 (28–43)	45 (35–56)	46 (35–58)
	Seminal vesicle (+)	—	2 (0–3)	6 (2–12)	5 (1–11)	9 (2–20)
	Lymph node (+)	—	1 (0–2)	4 (0–10)	6 (0–14)	6 (0–16)
2.6–4.0	Organ confined	80 (61–95)	63 (57–69)	41 (33–48)	30 (22–39)	25 (17–34)
	Extraprostatic extension	20 (5–39)	34 (28–40)	47 (40–55)	57 (47–67)	57 (46–68)
	Seminal vesicle (+)	—	2 (1–4)	9 (4–15)	7 (3–14)	12 (5–22)
	Lymph node (+)	—	1 (0–2)	3 (0–8)	4 (0–12)	5 (0–14)
4.1–6.0	Organ confined	75 (55–93)	57 (52–63)	35 (29–40)	25 (18–32)	21 (14–29)
	Extraprostatic extension	25 (7–45)	39 (33–44)	51 (44–57)	60 (50–68)	59 (49–69)
	Seminal vesicle (+)	—	2 (1–3)	7 (4–11)	5 (3–9)	9 (4–16)
	Lymph node (+)	—	2 (1–3)	7 (4–13)	10 (5–18)	10 (4–20)
6.1–10.0	Organ confined	69 (47–91)	49 (43–54)	26 (22–31)	19 (14–25)	15 (10–21)
	Extraprostatic extension	31 (9–53)	44 (39–49)	52 (46–58)	60 (52–68)	57 (48–67)
	Seminal vesicle (+)	—	5 (3–8)	16 (10–22)	13 (7–20)	19 (11–29)
	Lymph node (+)	—	2 (1–3)	6 (4–10)	8 (5–14)	8 (4–16)
>10.0	Organ confined	57 (35–86)	33 (28–38)	14 (11–17)	9 (6–13)	7 (4–10)
	Extraprostatic extension	43 (14–65)	52 (46–56)	47 (40–53)	50 (40–60)	46 (36–59)
	Seminal vesicle (+)	—	8 (5–11)	17 (12–24)	13 (8–21)	19 (12–29)
	Lymph node (+)	—	8 (5–12)	22 (15–30)	27 (16–39)	27 (14–40)

TABLE M-5.—Clinical Stage T2c (palpable on both lobes)

PSA Range (ng/mL)	Pathologic Stage	Gleason Score				
		2-4	5-6	3 + 4 = 7	4 + 3 = 7	8-10
0-2.5	Organ confined	86 (71-97)	73 (63-81)	51 (38-63)	39 (26-54)	34 (21-48)
	Extraprostatic extension	14 (3-29)	24 (17-33)	36 (26-48)	45 (32-59)	47 (33-61)
	Seminal vesicle (+)	—	1 (0-4)	5 (1-13)	5 (1-12)	8 (2-19)
	Lymph node (+)	—	1 (0-4)	6 (0-18)	9 (0-26)	10 (0-27)
2.6-4.0	Organ confined	78 (58-94)	61 (50-70)	38 (27-50)	27 (18-40)	23 (14-34)
	Extraprostatic extension	22 (6-42)	36 (27-45)	48 (37-59)	57 (44-70)	57 (44-70)
	Seminal vesicle (+)	—	2 (1-5)	8 (2-17)	6 (2-16)	10 (3-22)
	Lymph node (+)	—	1 (0-4)	5 (0-15)	7 (0-21)	8 (0-22)
4.1-6.0	Organ confined	73 (52-93)	55 (44-64)	31 (23-41)	21 (14-31)	18 (11-28)
	Extraprostatic extension	27 (7-48)	40 (32-50)	50 (40-60)	57 (43-68)	57 (43-70)
	Seminal vesicle (+)	—	2 (1-4)	6 (2-11)	4 (1-10)	7 (2-15)
	Lymph node (+)	—	3 (1-7)	12 (5-23)	16 (6-32)	16 (6-33)
6.1-10.0	Organ confined	67 (45-91)	46 (36-56)	24 (17-32)	16 (10-24)	13 (8-20)
	Extraprostatic extension	33 (9-55)	46 (37-55)	52 (42-61)	58 (46-69)	56 (43-69)
	Seminal vesicle (+)	—	5 (2-9)	13 (6-23)	11 (4-21)	16 (6-29)
	Lymph node (+)	—	3 (1-6)	10 (5-18)	13 (6-25)	13 (5-26)
>10.0	Organ confined	54 (32-85)	30 (21-38)	11 (7-17)	7 (4-12)	6 (3-10)
	Extraprostatic extension	46 (15-68)	51 (42-60)	42 (30-55)	43 (29-59)	41 (27-57)
	Seminal vesicle (+)	—	6 (2-12)	13 (6-24)	10 (3-20)	15 (5-28)
	Lymph node (+)	—	13 (6-22)	33 (18-49)	38 (20-58)	38 (20-59)

The disadvantages of Radical Prostatectomy:

▶ It is a major operation; the recovery period is six to eight weeks.

▶ There is a small risk of significant blood loss, so someone might want to donate blood for their surgery a month before in case a transfusion becomes necessary.

Potential postsurgical complications from prostatectomy include:

Sexual or Erectile Dysfunction. This generally occurs in at least 25% of men but it is a risk for everyone undergoing the operation. The degree of dysfunction is often related to age and the size of the cancer. Younger men and those with smaller tumors tend to have fewer sexual complications.

Incontinence (loss of urinary control). Urinary incontinence occurs in 3% to greater than 50% of men. In addition, it may take six to nine months to regain urinary control. In surveys that interviewed men one year after the operation, approximately 10% still reported some level of incontinence. Most often, this was related to stress incontinence (leakage of urine while straining—for example, swinging a golf club).

Bowel Complications. The number of men who experience rectal injury during surgery is less than 0.5%. If it should happen, the small defect can be fixed at the time of surgery with no long-term side effects.

▶ Preparing for Surgery: Things to Know

▶ Stop using any products that could cause blood to thin, such as aspirin and any dietary supplement, at least two weeks before surgery to prevent excessive bleeding during the operation.

▶ An enema or laxatives taken the night before surgery will assist with the elimination of fecal material. The rectum and part of the intestine need to be clear to reduce the chance of infection.

▶ A decision on the type of anesthesia used has to be made before surgery. There are two types of anesthesia: general anesthesia, which puts someone to sleep and is delivered in one dose; or epidural anesthesia, which numbs the area being operated on and can be delivered in more than one dose, according to individual needs. Although there have been some reports that epidural anesthesia reduces the risk of

Post-Operative Nomogram for Predicting Disease Recurrence After Surgery

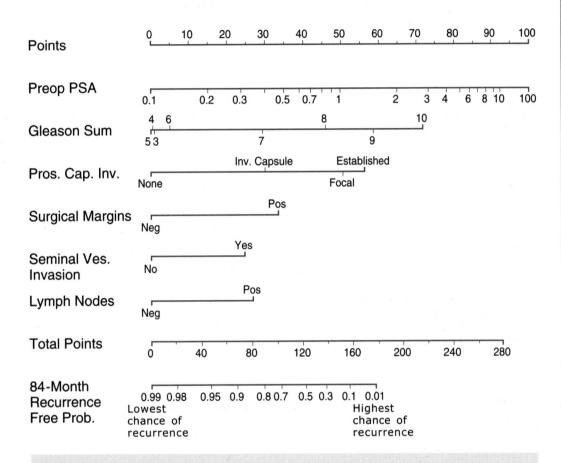

Instructions for Physician:
Locate the patient's PSA on the **PSA** axis. Draw a line straight upwards to the **Points** axis to determine how many points towards recurrence the patient receives for his PSA. Repeat this process for the other axes, each time drawing straight upward to the **Points** axis. Sum the points achieved for each predictor and locate this sum on the **Total Points** axis. Draw a line straight down to find the patient's probability of remaining recurrence free for 84 months assuming he does not die of another cause first.

Instruction to Patient:
"Mr. X, if we had 100 men exactly like you, we would expect between <predicted percentage from nomogram – 10%> and <predicted percentage + 10%> to remain free of their disease at 7 years following radical prostatectomy, and recurrence after 7 years is very rare."

developing blood clots in the legs, there has not been a formal study to prove or disprove this theory.

▶ If a man has had prior prostate surgery (as for BPH), he must wait two to three months between procedures. This allows time for the prostate to heal.

▶ Recovering from Surgery: What to Expect

In the hospital:

▶ The hospital stay will be two to seven days.

▶ After surgery there will be a catheter in the penis that drains urine from the bladder. This allows the urinary tract to rest and recover. The catheter must remain in place for two to three weeks.

▶ There will be one or two drainage tubes coming out of the lower abdomen that prevents internal fluid buildup or infection. The tubes will be in place for one to three days.

▶ Pain medication (Ketorolac® or Toradol®) will be given, which will relieve discomfort and help stimulate appetite within a few days.

▶ A laxative will be given to soften the stool, promote regular bowel movement, and prevent straining. (An enema should not be used for at least six weeks after surgery.)

At home:

▶ Do not lift anything heavier than ten pounds for six weeks after surgery.

▶ Do not drive a car for three weeks.

▶ Do not sit on a hard chair with a straight back for three weeks, or as long as the catheter is in place.

▶ There are no dietary restrictions.

▶ Walk regularly to prevent blood clots.

▶ Avoid any strenuous activity for at least six weeks after surgery.

EXTERNAL-BEAM RADIATION THERAPY

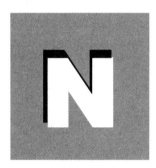

Over the past two decades, external-beam radiation therapy has been a common treatment for localized prostate cancer and the treatment of choice for locally-advanced cancer. External-beam radiation therapy is delivered from outside the body or from an external source, and includes:

► **3-DIMENSIONAL (3D) CONFORMAL BEAM RADIATION**

► **EXTERNAL-BEAM RADIATION**

► **EXTERNAL-BEAM RADIOTHERAPY**

► **NEUTRON BEAM RADIATION**

► **PROTON BEAM RADIATION**

► **RADICAL RADIATION**

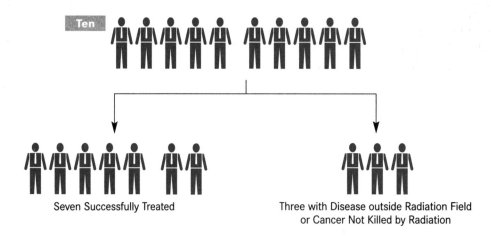

FIGURE N-1.—Radiation on any ten men.

Statistics	After 5 Years	After 10 Years	After 15 Years
TABLE N–1.—The Effectiveness of External-beam Radiation Therapy for Localized Prostate Cancer (T2)			
Percentage of men still alive (overall survival)	51–93%	41–70%	31–33%
Percentage of men who have not died of prostate cancer (disease-specific or cause-specific survival)	63–96%	66–86%	unknown
Percentage of men whose cancer has progressed (metastasis)	7–68%	36–60%	unknown

Note:
Cancer characteristics of these patients: 41% had well-differentiated, 41% had moderately differentiated, and 18% had poorly differentiated cancers.

Many institutions use a CT scan of the pelvis to accurately show technicians and doctors the exact location of the organs. A computer is then used to calculate the best possible positions the external beam can be targeted to most accurately deliver the radiation to the prostate. This is called 3-dimensional conformal beam radiation. During treatment, the individual lies on a table while the machine changes positions around the table. A variety of beam angles ensures the most effective treatment.

Men receive approximately 35 treatments over the course of 7 weeks, with weekends off. Each session takes 15 to 20 minutes and is painless. Radiation is targeted to specific

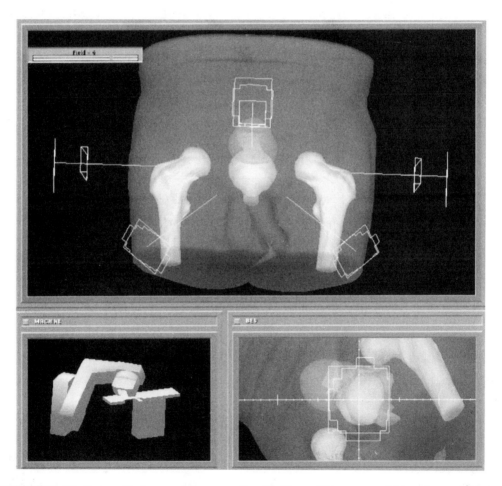

FIGURE N-2a.—External-beam Radiation Therapy Planning. These photographs show the computer model that determines the most effective radiation-beam angles for treatment.

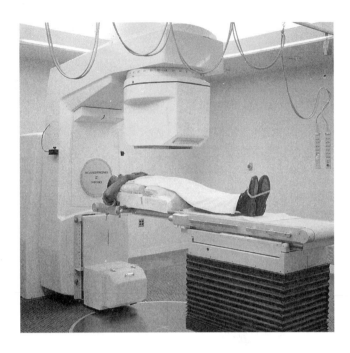

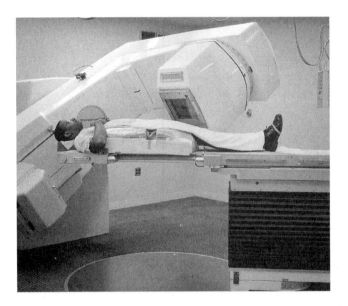

FIGURE N-2b.—External-beam Radiation Therapy Delivery. The actual delivery of external-beam radiation therapy from different angles. The treatment takes between 15 and 30 minutes per session.

3D Conformal Radiation Therapy Nomogram
for PSA Recurrence

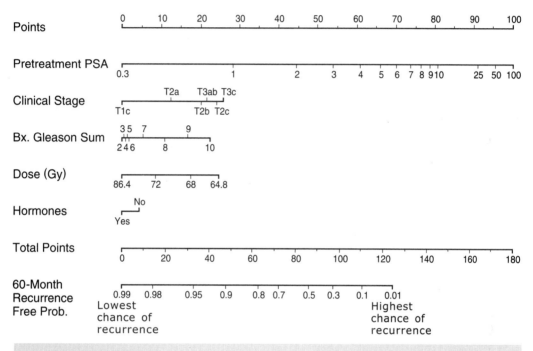

Instructions for Physician:

Locate the patient's PSA on the **PSA** axis. Draw a line straight upwards to the **Points** axis to determine how many points towards recurrence the patient receives for his PSA. Repeat this process for the other axes, each time drawing straight upward to the **Points** axis. Sum the points achieved for each predictor and locate this sum on the **Total Points** axis. Draw a line straight down to find the patient's probability of remaining recurrence free for 60 months assuming he does not die of another cause first.

Note: This nomogram is not applicable to a a man who is not otherwise a candidate for radiation therapy. You can use this only on a man who has already selected radiation therapy as treatment for his prostate cancer.

Instruction to Patient:

"Mr. X, if we had 100 men exactly like you, we would expect between <predicted percentage from nomogram – 10%> and <predicted percentage + 10%> to remain free of their disease at 7 years following radical prostatectomy, and recurrence after 7 years is very rare."

areas and does not reach areas that do not need it. Lead blocks protect those sites. Regardless of whether the cancer has spread beyond the prostate, radiation is given to the areas immediately surrounding the prostate.

Radiation therapy can be used for men of any age with any stage of cancer.

Therefore, the best candidates for this treatment are:

▶ Men who are expected to live at least 10 more years.

▶ Men whose cancer is confined to the prostate.

▶ Men who cannot be cured by surgery because the cancer has escaped the prostate but is still thought to be nearby (men with stage T3 cancer).

▶ Men whose cancer has returned after initial surgical treatment.

▶ Men who do not want to be treated with surgery.

As for surgery, nomograms have been developed to help predict if external beam radiation will be successful in controlling the cancer (page 135). Control is measured in terms of men being free of a PSA recurrence.

The advantages of radiation therapy:

▶ The outcome for men with localized cancer is similar to that of radical prostatectomy (surgical removal of the prostate). Between 40% and 60% of men with both localized and advanced cancer are alive 15 years after treatment.

▶ It is done on an outpatient basis.

The disadvantages of radiation therapy:

▶ It is difficult afterward for doctors to tell if someone has been cured, because a low PSA level after radiation therapy does not always guarantee total elimination of the cancer.

▶ The cancer cannot be pathologically staged (the prostate is not removed, so it cannot be examined by a pathologist).

▶ There are complications associated with radiation therapy. Side effects usually develop toward the end of the treatment, or even months after the therapy has ended.

▶ It is expensive, with an average total cost of between $10,000 and $30,000.

▶ Neutron and Proton Radiation

Like an X-ray, standard radiation uses high-energy photons that pass through the body, imparting energy to anything in the path of the beam. The power in the beam itself decreases as it goes through the body, leaving most of its energy in the first tissues or area it hits. As a result, standard radiation is most useful for cancers near the surface of the body. The deeper inside the body the cancer is (like prostate cancer), the stronger the beam needed to get to it, and the larger the dose of radiation the healthy tissue absorbs, which increases unwanted side effects.

Neutron and proton radiation are relatively new treatments, but they have been approved by the FDA and are covered by Medicare and most other health insurance companies.

Like standard radiation, these therapies are most effective for cancers lying close to the body surface. Neutron and proton therapies use particles (neutrons and protons) that have different qualities than the photons used in standard therapy. For example, they only go a limited distance into the body, rather than passing through, and that distance can be determined by the starting energy of the particle. The greater the starting energy, the farther into the body it goes. Also, the amount of energy neutrons and protons deliver increases as they slow down, and they give off a large burst of energy when they stop. So unlike standard radiation therapy, where the maximum dose is found at the surface, in neutron and proton treatment, the maximum dose can be placed inside the cancer itself, decreasing the damage to the healthy tissue of the body. This allows the delivery of far greater doses of radiation to the cancer without an increase in side effects.

Photons
(No Charge and Mass)

Neutrons
(Negative Charge with Mass)

Protons
(Positive Charge with Mass)

FIGURE N-3.—Radiation particle symbols.

Neutron Radiation

Today, there are only a few places in the United States that perform neutron therapy, but in the future, more institutions may offer it as an option.

The usual period of treatment with neutron radiation is one to two months, with treatments given Monday through Friday for 15 to 30 minutes. Treatment is similar to regular external-beam radiation where someone lies on a table and radiation beams are aimed at them. These treatments are painless.

Proton Radiation

Proton radiation's ability to specifically target a dose to the cancer has been useful for treating eye, brain, and spine cancers, where damage to the surrounding area can be very dangerous. However, there have not been many clinical trials of this treatment that involve other areas of the body. Currently, Massachusetts General Hospital in Boston and Loma Linda University Medical Center in Loma Linda, California, are working together on clinical trials of proton radiation and prostate cancer.

Hormonal Ablation and Radiation Therapy

When hormonal ablation is used in conjunction with radiation therapy, it may increase the effectiveness of treatment. It can be given in the neoadjuvant setting (prior to the start of radiation), the concurrent setting (during radiation), and the adjuvant setting (after radiation). Why would hormonal ablation help?

There are a number of possibilities:

▶ It may reduce the number of cancer cells that have to be eliminated by radiation.

▶ Apoptosis, or cell death, may be enhanced.

▶ It may cause cancer cells to be more dependent on oxygen, and also make them more likely to be killed by radiation (photon radiation is better at killing cancer cells that depend on oxygen).

▶ It may cause cancer cells to stop dividing and to stop reproducing so that the cancer is more likely to be killed by radiation.

Neoadjuvant and Concurrent Therapy. A study done in the 1970s using DES (an estrogen) prior to radiation therapy for locally-advanced cancers showed an almost 20% higher rate of local control, compared to radiation therapy alone. Other studies using other hormones (LHRH agonist and an antiandrogen) before and during radiation therapy found 25% better control rates for cancer than radiation therapy alone.

However, the best length of time to use hormonal therapy in conjunction with radiation therapy is not yet known. Some studies are now extending neoadjuvant therapy from three months to eight months before therapy, and the early findings seem to suggest improved results for men undergoing longer therapy. Most of these studies keep the man on hormone ablation while radiation therapy is given.

Concurrent and Adjuvant Therapy. In 1998, a study showed that men with T3 and T4 prostate cancer may keep cancer away longer and live longer if they are given hormonal ablation as soon as radiation therapy is started, and then for three years after treatment. In this study, about 80% of the men receiving combined treatment were alive five years after treatment, versus a little more than 60% of the men receiving only radiation. In addition, of the men who were alive after five years, 85% had no signs of disease, versus 48% of those who only received radiation.

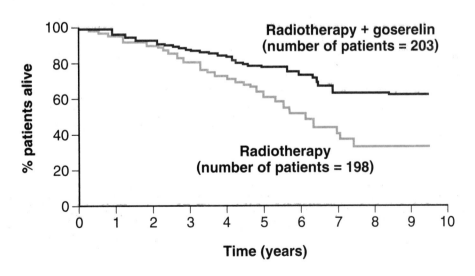

FIGURE N-4.—Probability of overall survival over a 10-year period following treatment with radiotherapy plus goserelin compared with radiation therapy alone.

This appears to be great news for men with locally-advanced prostate cancer, but more research is needed. Also, there are some things to remember when considering these results. For example:

▶ The men in the study were either given radiation therapy or radiation therapy in combination with hormonal ablation. There were no men in the study who received hormonal ablation alone. It could be that men will do just as well on hormonal ablation with no other treatment.

▶ The study only followed men for about four years—the rest of the data was based on estimates.

▶ Men who were given the combined treatment experienced more incontinence (about 30% versus about 15%), and naturally experienced hormonal ablation-related side effects such as hot flashes (in about 60% of the men).

Generally, it is now recommended that men with high risk localized prostate cancer or men with locally-advanced prostate cancer receive two to three years of hormone therapy in conjunction with radiation therapy. This includes men that have:

▶ T2 cancer with Gleason score 8–10.

▶ T2 cancer with PSA ≥ 20 at diagnosis.

▶ T2 cancer with PSA 10–20 and Gleason score 7 at diagnosis.

▶ T3 cancer, with any PSA and Gleason score.

▶ Complications Associated with Radiation Therapy (from most to least common)

Sexual or Erectile Dysfunction

The majority of men who receive radiation therapy do not have problems with erections or sexual activity in the short term. However, depending on the study, 30% or more of men receiving radiation therapy can have some sexual complications in the long run. Because some of the best candidates for radiation therapy are older men, and some degree of sexual dysfunction happens with increased age, it is hard to say exactly how strongly radiation affects sexual function.

Bowel Complications

Diarrhea, rectal pain, and the feeling of constantly wanting to have a bowel movement are the most common bowel complications associated with radiation therapy. However, in large studies involving more than 1,000 men receiving radiation therapy, the incidence of chronic bowel complications was approximately 5%. A very low percentage of men have occasional, painless rectal bleeding after radiation treatments. This has been likened to what people experience when they have hemorrhoids.

Urinary Problems

A man may leak urine, need to urinate often (especially at night), feel the urge to constantly urinate, or experience painful urination while undergoing radiation therapy. Studies have shown that more than three out of four men (75%) who undergo radiation therapy will need some type of medication to help with urination while they are receiving treatment. However, less than 5% of men who undergo radiation therapy experience urinary complications serious enough to require hospitalization. Less than 1% of those hospitalized require an operation to fix the problem.

The most common complaints among people undergoing radiation therapy are having to urinate more often and/or having blood in the urine. Complications requiring hospitalization include urethral strictures (narrowing or blockage of the urethra from scar tissue), bladder problems, and/or bloody urine. The majority of such hospitalizations are among men who have had surgery for benign prostate enlargement prior to undergoing treatment for prostate cancer. Overall, approximately 5% will experience long-term complications, which is very similar to that reported for surgery patients.

BRACHYTHERAPY

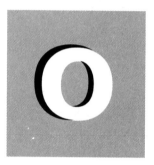

Another type of radiation therapy can be delivered from inside the body from an internal source. This can be called:

> ▶ **BRACHYTHERAPY**
> ▶ **INTERSTITIAL RADIOTHERAPY**
> ▶ **INTERSTITIAL SEED IMPLANTS**
> ▶ **PERMANENT SEED IMPLANTS**
> ▶ **RADIOACTIVE SEED IMPLANTS**
> ▶ **SEED IMPLANTS**
> ▶ **TEMPORARY SEED IMPLANTS**

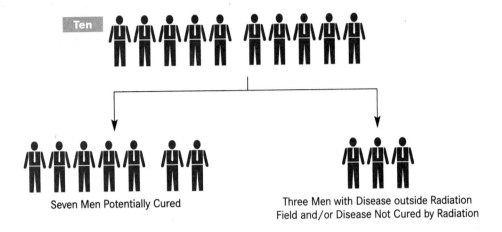

Seven Men Potentially Cured

Three Men with Disease outside Radiation Field and/or Disease Not Cured by Radiation

FIGURE O-1.—Seed implants plus radiation statistics.

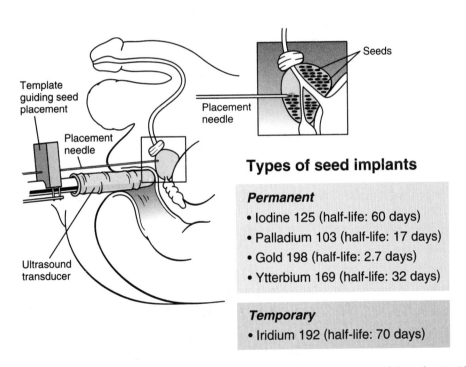

Template guiding seed placement

Placement needle

Placement needle

Ultrasound transducer

Seeds

Types of seed implants

Permanent
- Iodine 125 (half-life: 60 days)
- Palladium 103 (half-life: 17 days)
- Gold 198 (half-life: 2.7 days)
- Ytterbium 169 (half-life: 32 days)

Temporary
- Iridium 192 (half-life: 70 days)

FIGURE O-2.—A side view of permanent radioactive-seed implantation performed under the guidence of transrectal ultrasound, or TRUS. Small box: the various types of radioactive seeds used, the most popular of which are Palladium 103 and Iodine 125.

Radiation therapy that is delivered internally to fight prostate cancer uses many small "seeds" (each about the size of a grain of rice) of radioactive material that are implanted directly into the prostate gland. The radioactive seeds (usually either Iodine 125 or Palladium 103) are placed inside the prostate tissue, hence the word "interstitial," which means "situated within." The prefix "brachy" means "short," so the concept is to implant the radioactive seeds within the prostate a short distance from the cancer, where they should be the most effective. The general idea is that radiation is delivered directly inside the prostate as opposed to traveling from the outside in. Some types of seeds remain permanently in place, while others are later removed.

Before the seeds are implanted in the prostate, a great deal of time is spent understanding exactly where the cancer is and the precise location of the prostate. Doctors want to know exactly where to place the radioactive seeds and how much radiation the seeds should give off. This will vary from man to man because the location and aggressiveness of a cancer can be different from one individual to the next. In general, the higher the grade of cancer, the higher the dose of radiation, or isotope, used. Iodine 125 seeds may be best for slow-growing, low-grade cancers, while Palladium 103 and the temporary seed implant Iridium 192 may be best for faster-growing, high-grade cancers. The higher the radiation dosage, the more effective the treatment, but the greater the severity of side effects.

For at least 10 days before the procedure, blood-thinning products such as aspirin must be discontinued to prevent excess bleeding during the procedure. The night before the procedure, an enema must be used to empty the rectum, and no food or liquids are allowed until the procedure is over.

▶ Permanent Radioactive Seed Implantation

Once the exact location of the prostate is determined through X-ray or ultrasound, between 70 and 150 seeds are implanted throughout the prostate via thin needles passed through the skin of the perineum (the area between the testicles and the anus). The number of seeds used depends on the size of the prostate. An ultrasound probe is inserted into the rectum to help the surgeon determine the proper placement of the seeds.

The procedure is performed under spinal anesthesia and lasts about 45 minutes to an hour. After the procedure a catheter is placed until the numbness wears off, which takes about two hours. Driving is prohibited for the first 12 hours, and strenuous activity should be avoided for 48 hours. After two to three days, normal activities can be resumed. Although this type of radiation probably does not escape the prostate, for the first couple of months it is recommended that those with implants should stay at least six feet away from

Pretreatment Nomogram for Predicting Freedom from Recurrence After Permanent Prostate Brachytherapy in Prostate Cancer

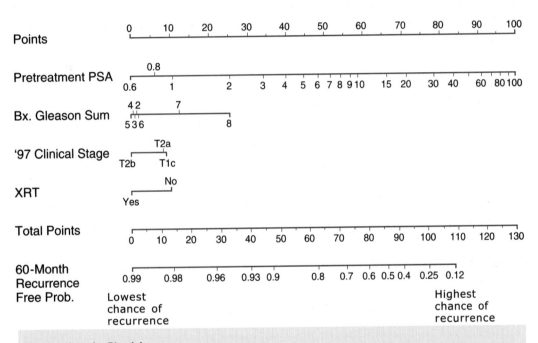

Instructions for Physician:
Locate the patient's PSA on the **Pretreatment PSA** axis. Draw a line straight upwards to the **Points** axis to determine how many points towards recurrence the patient receives for his PSA. Repeat this process for the other axes, each time drawing straight upward to the **Points** axis. Sum the points achieved for each predictor and locate this sum on the **Total Points** axis. Draw a line straight down to find the patient's probability of remaining recurrence free for 60 months assuming he does not die of another cause first.

Note: This nomogram is not applicable to a man who is not otherwise a candidate for permanent prostate brachytherapy. You can use this only on a man who has already selected permanent prostate brachytherapy as treatment for his prostate cancer. You must decide upon use of adjuvant XRT prior to consulting this nomogram.

Instruction to Patient:
"Mr. X, if we had 100 men exactly like you, we would expect between <predicted percentage from nomogram – 30%> and <predicted percentage + 5%> to remain free of their disease at 5 years following permanent prostate brachytherapy, and recurrence after 5 years is very rare."

pregnant women and children, who are most sensitive to radiation. The radioactivity itself is usually gone after one year.

Nomograms have been developed to help predict how well brachytherapy may work for patients based on clinical stage, pre-treatment PSA, Gleason Score, and whether external beam radiation therapy is also given (page 145).

The best candidates for permanent radioactive-seed implantation are:

▶ Men with localized prostate cancer (stages T1 or T2; A or B) who have a life expectancy of at least 10 years.

▶ Older men (70 and above) with localized prostate cancer who are not candidates for surgery due to other medical conditions.

The advantages of permanent seed implantation:

▶ Results indicate that it is as effective as external-beam radiation or surgery in the short term (up to five years).

▶ In some cases there is no need for additional external beam radiation therapy.

▶ Seed implants deliver about twice the effective dose of radiation to the prostate versus that of external-beam radiation alone.

▶ The procedure is relatively noninvasive.

▶ There is minimal effect on urinary control and minimal associated bleeding.

▶ It is a new technique, so its effectiveness may continue to improve.

▶ It is covered by Medicare and other forms of insurance.

The disadvantages of permanent seed implantation:

▶ Long-term (10- and 15-year) results of the newer and more effective transperineal procedure, combined with external-beam radiation, are not yet available.

▶ Most long-term data collected to date are from only a few institutions.

▶ Complications include difficulty urinating, rectal discomfort, sexual dysfunction, and swelling or inflammation of the prostate.

▶ After undergoing this procedure, a man is usually no longer a candidate for surgery.

▶ It is expensive, with a total average cost of $15,000 to $25,000.

▶ **Temporary Radioactive Seed Implantation**

This procedure, also called "iridium template therapy," "high-dose-rate (HDR) brachytherapy," and "fractionated HDR conformal prostate brachytherapy" is a little different from the standard ultrasound-guided permanent seed implant procedure and requires a short stay in the hospital. It involves placing an intense radiation source directly into or around the cancer for a short period of time. After the man receives a spinal anesthetic, 12–20 small, flexible plastic needles are inserted through the perineum and into the prostate. This is done under ultrasound guidance, and the procedure itself takes about one and a half hours. A small plastic plate, which holds the needles in place, is left next to the perineum. A bladder catheter inserted during the procedure is also kept in place until the next day.

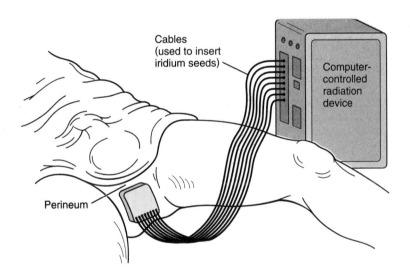

FIGURE O-3.—Temporary radioactive-seed implantation: Iridium seeds (also called "bars") are inserted and timed using a computer-controlled radiation device.

Radiation treatment planning, based on a CT scan of the prostate, begins after the needles are inserted. After the strategy is approved, the individual receives the first of three high-dose-radiation (HDR) treatments. An HDR machine under computer control transfers an intense radioactive source to each implanted needle. The treatment takes five to eight minutes and is painless. The remaining two treatments are given the next day, in the morning and afternoon. After the last HDR treatment, the template, needles, and bladder catheter are removed. Once the man is able to urinate, he is able to leave the hospital. He should spend a quiet evening at home and the next day a radiation oncologist or urologist will meet with him to examine the perineum.

The second phase of treatment involves external-beam radiation therapy (usually about two weeks later). This typically involves 20 individual external-beam radiation treatments given daily, Monday through Friday, for four weeks.

The short-term side effects of temporary seed implants include:

▶ Urinary frequency and burning

▶ Rectal irritation

▶ Intestinal gas

▶ Soft bowel movements

▶ Mild fatigue

The advantages of temporary seed implants:

▶ Between 60% and 80% of those who are fully potent before the procedure will remain potent afterward. Any symptoms of impotence are usually temporary.

▶ Most men continue to work full time during the follow-up external-beam radiation therapy.

▶ The three-year disease-free survival rate is 85%.

The disadvantages of temporary seed implants:

▶ About 5% of patients experience minor urethral strictures (narrowing of the urethra with scar tissue), which may require treatment.

▶ Men who have had a previous transurethral resection of the prostate (TURP), usually do not qualify for the procedure.

▶ The procedure is expensive, costing 35% to 50% more than a standard ultrasound-guided seed-implant procedure.

▶ This is a very new procedure, so there are no long-term data on its effectiveness.

The complication rate, time involved, pain, and cost are lower with the permanent seed implant procedure versus that of the temporary iridium template procedure. However, early results suggest that it may be as effective as permanent seed implantation.

CRYOTHERAPY

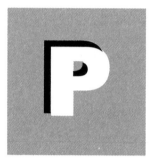

Cryotherapy is the medical term for freezing the prostate. The prefix "cryo" means "to freeze," and the word "ablation" means "to get rid of." So, prostatic cryoablation means to get rid of the prostate cancer by freezing it. Also called cryotherapy or cryosurgery, this is not performed by very many doctors. For awhile, many doctors were trying this therapy, but it has not been proven to be very popular. However, it is still a unique approach for treating prostate cancer that merits discussion.

During this transrectal ultrasound-guided procedure (performed under general or regional anesthesia), very cold liquid nitrogen (the same kind used in fire extinguishers) is used to freeze the prostate. Five small punctures are made in the perineum (the area between the testicles and anus), through which five metallic probes, or rods, are inserted. Liquid nitrogen is delivered through these rods into the prostate. The five thin metallic probes, each roughly 6 inches long, deliver temperatures of –185°C to –195°C into the prostate until it becomes, quite literally, an "iceball."

Afterward, the frozen cancerous area melts. During thawing, the cancer cells break apart, or burst. Although the prostate itself is frozen during the procedure, the urethra (the urinary tract that runs through the gland) is kept warm with a special warming device so that it is not damaged.

Cryotherapy takes two to three hours. This procedure can be uncomfortable, but anesthesia is given so that it is well tolerated. The man either goes home that day or stays overnight in the hospital. Medication is given for any discomfort, and Hytrin® or Cardura® (medications that relax the prostate) help reduce swelling for several weeks after the procedure. Men also take antibiotics for several days after the procedure, and a catheter and/or abdominal tube (called a suprapubic tube) must be used for two to three weeks until the swelling goes down and normal urination returns.

The best candidates for cryotherapy are:

▶ Older men (age 70 or above) with stage T1 or T2 prostate cancer.

▶ Men who do not qualify for surgery or radiation therapy.

▶ Men who do not want surgery or radiation therapy.

▶ Men who have failed radiation therapy.

The advantages of cryotherapy:

▶ It only requires a short hospital stay, if any.

▶ It is a relatively noninvasive procedure.

The disadvantages of cryotherapy:

▶ Impotence. About 9 out of 10 men (90%) experience long-term difficulties in having erections (ask your doctor about newer cryotherapy procedures that allow for nerve sparing).

▶ Short-term urinary problems. Most men will have problems urinating for several weeks after the procedure because the prostate enlarges temporarily and presses on the urethra, or urinary tract, cutting off the flow of urine.

▶ The long-term effectiveness and side effects of this procedure are not known.

▶ Cryosurgery is expensive. The total average cost is $13,000–$15,000, and many insurance companies do not cover it.

TREATMENTS FOR INCONTINENCE AND IMPOTENCE

▶ The Most Common Side Effects of Local Therapy

Urinary Incontinence

Incontinence, or loss of urinary control, is also known as bed wetting, leakage, and dribbling. It is a common problem in men and women. Incontinence affects more than 10 million Americans, but less than 10% seek medical attention. However, it is estimated that Americans spend $15 billion a year in the quest to stay dry.

Incontinence can occur for a number of reasons, including age and physical stress, such as lifting. Treatment for prostate cancer (radical prostatectomy and radiation therapy) can also lead to incontinence. Among men who undergo surgery for prostate cancer, in most cases the condition is temporary and resolves itself over time or can be corrected with minor treatment. However, less than 5% of prostatectomy and radiation patients experience severe incontinence that can only be corrected with surgery.

Regardless of the severity, the problem is usually treatable. However, it must first be diagnosed with one or more of the following tests:

Cystogram. A test in which a tube (called a catheter) is placed through the penis into the bladder. Through this tube, the bladder is slowly filled with a type of dye that allows the doctor to view the organ upon X-ray.

Cystometrogram. A test in which a catheter is used to measure and record the bladder's average pressure as it fills with and releases urine.

Cystoscopy. A procedure in which a lighted tube (called a cystoscope) is guided up the penis and into the bladder so the doctor can see how well the continence-controlling muscles work.

Urinary Flow Rate. A test that measures the speed with which the urine leaves the penis (in milliliters per second, or ml/sec).

Urine Culture. This is when a urine sample is analyzed for bacteria that could be causing an infection, a possible explanation for urinary trouble.

There are basically five types of incontinence, all of which can be caused by prostate cancer treatment. These types of incontinence can occur separately or together:

Overflow Incontinence ~ (also called) False Incontinence. This is when the bladder never drains completely because the urethra and/or bladder neck is scarred and narrowed, or the bladder no longer contracts due to certain medications or injury. Therefore, the bladder is constantly filling with urine and the pressure becomes too great, which causes leakage. Typical symptoms of overflow incontinence include:

▶ Being unable to urinate even though when feeling the urge.
▶ Getting up repeatedly at night to urinate.
▶ Leaking small amounts of urine throughout the day.
▶ Taking a long time to urinate and when it finally happens, the stream may be very weak.
▶ Feeling like the bladder is still full even after urinating.

Stress Incontinence ~ (also called) Anatomic Incontinence.   This is when any movement or action that could put pressure on the bladder results in urine leakage. Symptoms include:

▶   Leaking urine when coughing, laughing, sneezing, or exercising.

▶   Leaking urine on standing from a seated position or getting out of bed.

▶   Needing to urinate more often so the bladder is never too full.

Urge Incontinence.   This is when the urge to urinate is so great someone cannot "hold it." This occurs because the bladder is pushing urine out with so much force that its sphincter cannot hold it back. Symptoms include:

▶   Getting up many times at night to urinate

▶   Needing to urinate every few hours throughout the day

▶   Wetting the bed at night or wetting oneself on the way to the bathroom

Total Incontinence.   This is when the bladder constantly leaks urine, regardless of the time of day or what type of activity.

Mixed Incontinence.   This is when two or more types of incontinence occur together, such as stress and urge incontinence.

Absorbent male undergarments, or adult diapers, are effective in managing leakage and are usually used as the first line of defense for those who leak in the initial months after surgery or radiation therapy. They are relatively inexpensive, save a lot of potential embarrassment and expense from soiled clothing and furniture, and most are not noticeable under clothing. There are basically four types of disposable or reusable products that absorb urine effectively:

Adult Undergarments.   These are the bulkiest of the protective undergarments, and they look like heavily padded underwear. They are usually worn only at night or while at home.

Adult Briefs.   These are less bulky than undergarments and can be worn like underwear under loose clothing.

Adult Pads. These are pads that come in all degrees of thickness and are placed inside regular underwear. They can be worn without notice under regular clothing.

Bed or Mattress Pads. These cover and protect a bed or mattress.

To prevent or lessen the severity of incontinence, some physicians have men do Kegel exercises (also called special perineal exercises) before and after prostate surgery. These exercises involve strengthening the pelvic muscles by deliberately starting and stopping the urine flow. When not urinating, the same results can be achieved by tightening the muscles of the pelvis or buttocks. Regular practice of the Kegel exercises may reduce leakage or correct it permanently. These exercises should be repeated three times a day for several weeks or months. Results vary from individual to individual; some think they can cure incontinence with these exercises while others think they are useless.

There are two sets of muscles, or sphincters, that prevent urinary leakage: those at the base of the bladder (also called bladder-neck muscles or the internal sphincter) and those directly below the bladder (also called the external sphincter) that surround the urethra (the tube that carries urine from the body). If anything happens to these muscles or the nerves that control them, incontinence can result.

Radiation therapy causes long-term (greater than one year after treatment) urinary incontinence in less than 5% of men treated. This type of incontinence usually occurs after the treatment has been completed. If radiation therapy damages the sphincter muscles that prevent urine leakage, the result is stress incontinence. If the radiation affects the bladder as a whole, the resulting irritation can cause urge incontinence. If both structures are affected by radiation, then both types of incontinence are likely to occur (mixed incontinence).

Radical prostatectomy causes long-term (greater than one year after treatment) urinary incontinence in 3% to greater than 50% of men. The reason for this wide variation is because the surgeon performing the operation has a lot to do with the incontinence risk. However, incontinence after the surgery is not 100% dependent on the surgeon. Incontinence will result in a small percentage of men regardless of the surgeon's skill. However, it is very important to choose an experienced surgeon—one who has not only performed this surgery many times but who continues to perform it regularly (at least four times a month).

Cryosurgery, in which the prostate gland is frozen, can also cause freezing of the urinary sphincter, resulting in long-term incontinence in 5% to 15% of men.

▶ Nonsurgical Treatment of Incontinence

There are a number of medications and nonsurgical procedures that may help incontinence:

Ditropan® (oxybutinin). This is one of the most popular incontinence medications (an anticholinergic drug). The dosage is 2.5 or 5 mg two to four times a day, depending on how well the medication is tolerated. The potential side effects are usually dry mouth, drowsiness, and heart palpitations. It should not be given to people with increased eye (intraocular) pressure (glaucoma).

Pro-Banthine® (propantheline bromide). This drug is usually not as effective as Ditropan but can be used along with it, and a few men find it easier to tolerate. The regular dosage is 15 mg two to three times a day. Some men take a larger dose at bedtime to prevent leakage while they sleep. The potential side effects include dry mouth, visual problems, and glaucoma.

Tofranil® (imipramine hydrochloride). This drug is very effective in controlling leakage. The dosage is 10 or 25 mg two to four times daily. The potential side effects are dry mouth, constipation, blurred vision, and feeling tired or sleepy.

Chlorpheniramine Maleate®. A widely used antihistamine that is available in long-working 8-mg capsules taken once a day or 4-mg capsules taken twice a day. It can also be taken with another medication called Ornade Spansules. Side effects are dry nasal passages and a dry mouth.

Muscle Relaxants. Drugs such as flavoxate hydrochloride (Urispas®) can be taken orally (200 mg) three to four times a day.

Catheterization ~ (also called) Self-Catheterization. Some men whose bladders cannot generate a forceful contraction to urinate can be treated by regular or occasional self-catheterization. When performing self-catheterization, a small, narrow tube called a catheter is placed inside the penis every four to six hours to drain the bladder of urine. This always sounds more difficult than it is, but after a few times most men are very comfortable using a catheter. Men who carry their catheters with them can enjoy a wide range of normal activities.

Condom Catheters and Penile Clamps. The condom catheter is a condom that is placed over the penis that drains any leaked urine into a bag. A penile clamp is a device that literally clamps the penis, closing the urethra from the outside to prevent urine leakage. Neither device should be used as a first-line treatment. The condom catheter can cause numerous infections, while the penile clamp can scar or damage the penis.

► Surgical Treatment of Incontinence

Surgical treatment of incontinence should only be considered for men whose leakage is extreme, lasting at least a year without signs of improvement. There are two surgical options for incontinence: transurethral collagen injection and artificial urinary sphincter.

► Transurethral Collagen Injection

Collagen is a protein found throughout the human body. Many people have already received collagen injections to fill in scars or wrinkles. The collagen used in this procedure is derived from cows.

This minimally invasive outpatient treatment can be performed under local anesthesia. During the procedure, a cystoscope is placed into the penis and guided up into the bladder through which collagen is injected into the bladder neck. The addition of collagen closes the opening of the bladder into the urethra, but this opening expands normally during voluntary urination.

Three to four treatments are usually required before a successful result may be achieved. Because each injection costs several hundred dollars, it is not unusual for this treatment to cost several thousand dollars.

It is important to wait at least a year after prostate surgery before considering collagen injections to make sure that the incontinence has had an ample chance to improve on its own. It is also important to have a skin test about a month before the surgery to rule out the chance of an allergic reaction to the collagen. During a skin test, a small amount of collagen is injected into the skin of the arm to see if any redness, swelling, or itching occurs that would indicate a possible sensitivity. This usually occurs in the first three days, but it can happen for up to a month. Such an allergy is extremely rare, affecting less than 1% of men.

Men who experience incontinence from radiation treatment are not good candidates for collagen injections, as scar tissue caused by the radiation prevents the material from

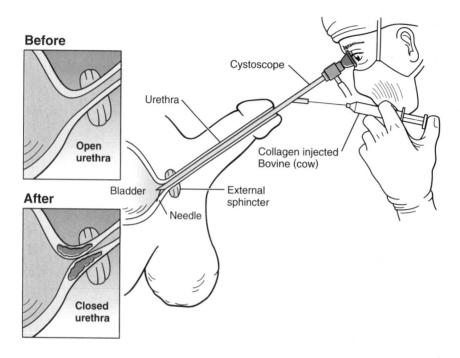

Before

Open
urethra

After

Closed
urethra

Cystoscope

Urethra

Collagen injected
Bovine (cow)

Bladder

External
sphincter

Needle

FIGURE Q-1.—During the Transurethral Collagen injection procedure, a cystoscope is placed into the penis and up into the bladder, through which collagen is injected into the bladder neck. The addition of collagen closed the opening of the bladder into the urethra, which prevents urin leakage, however, the urethra expands normally upon voluntary urination.

being injected properly. Among men whose leakage is caused by surgery, collagen treatment works well in about a third of those who request it. It may work well for several months or many years—the results vary from person to person.

The best candidates for collagen implants are:

▶ Men with minimal incontinence (who use one to two pads daily) who have not shown improvement in their symptoms for at least a year after treatment.

▶ Men whose incontinence has been caused by surgery.

The advantages of collagen injection:

▶ The procedure is done on an outpatient basis.

▶ The collagen works naturally and there is nothing else the man has to do.

The disadvantages of collagen injection:

▶ It is not effective in men whose incontinence has been caused by radiation therapy.

▶ The treatment process requires multiple injections/sessions.

▶ The long-term effectiveness (after two years) is not known.

▶ The injections are expensive, with a total cost of between $2,000 and $10,000.

▶ Artificial Urinary Sphincter

This is a surgically implanted device that can be used to correct severe, long-term incontinence that has lasted a year or more. It consists of a cuff placed around the urethra or bladder neck. When the cuff is inflated with saline solution (manually triggered by a pump implanted in the scrotum), it squeezes shut the urethra or bladder neck and thus prevents urine leakage. When the cuff is deflated, the pressure is released and urination can occur.

While complications from this device are rare, they can include infection, continued urine leakage, bleeding, and mechanical malfunction. The artificial sphincter can be implanted successfully in 95% of cases.

The operation is performed under spinal or general anesthesia and requires a one- or two-day hospital stay. Two incisions are made, the first is below the scrotum and the second is in the lower abdominal area. After surgery, a catheter may be inserted to drain the bladder, but it is usually removed before someone leaves the hospital. A drainage tube may also be placed in the abdomen if there is excess fluid near the incision site.

The artificial sphincter itself cannot be used for four to six weeks after surgery, because the urethra needs this time to recover. Therefore, the individual remains incontinent during this period. Following the recovery period, the doctor activates the artificial sphincter, after which it can be manually controlled. The artificial sphincter is made from a type of rubber called silicone elastomer, which is not a silicone gel. There is no evidence that this type of silicone causes an allergic reaction.

The best candidates for artificial sphincters are men with severe incontinence (who use three pads or more daily) whose symptoms have not improved for at least a year.

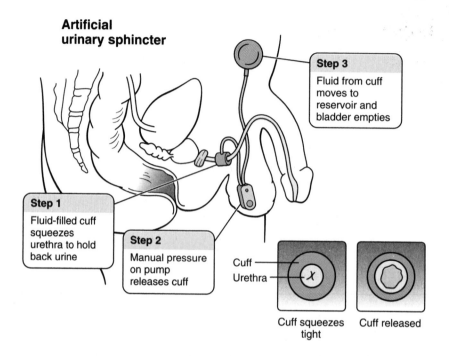

FIGURE Q-2.—The Artificial Urinary Sphincter consists of a cuff that is placed around the urethra or bladder neck. When the cuff is inflated with saline (manually triggered by a pump implanted in the scrotum), it squeezes shut the urethra or bladder neck, thus blocking urine flow. When the cuff is deflated, the pressure on the urinary tract is released and urination can occur.

The advantages of the artificial urinary sphincter:

▶ It is the most effective treatment for severe, long-term incontinence.

▶ It is easy to use.

The disadvantages of the artificial urinary sphincter:

▶ There is a long-term risk of mechanical failure, requiring replacement.

▶ It requires a one- to two-day hospital stay.

▶ It is expensive, costing an average total of $12,000 to $18,000.

▶ Erectile Dysfunction

Erectile dysfunction means that a man has trouble with erection. He may not be able to stay erect very long, he may not be able to achieve an erection every time, or his erections may not be as strong as they were before treatment.

Treatments for Erectile Dysfunction

There are a variety of interventions for men whose erectile dysfunction is associated with prostate-cancer treatment. They include:

Viagra® (sildenafil citrate). This medication is used for erectile dysfunction. It comes in 25 mg, 50 mg, and 100 mg tablets. It should be taken approximately 1 hour before sexual stimulation. In most men with nerve bundles to the penis, it has been shown to improve the quality of erections. In some men after surgery and radiation therapy, it can improve the quality of erections. This medicine should not be used without doctor supervision. It also should not be used by men who have had a heart attack within the last 6 months, or who have chest pain or low blood pressure. Other medicines similar to sildenafil are being developed and may be approved soon to help improve the quality of erections.

New Oral Treatments for Erectile Dysfunction. Ask your doctor about these medications because several of these may be approved in the next year or two (apomorphine, tadalafil, vardenafil, . . .).

Penile Self-Injections. This involves using a tiny needle and syringe to self-inject medication into the side of the penis. The drug causes blood to flow into the areas of the penis called the corpus cavernosa and the corpus spongiosum, which produces a strong erection. Men are usually surprised at how simple and painless this can be.

The medications used include one or more of the following: phentolamine, papaverine or prostaglandin E (PGE). Men learn from their doctor how inject the medication properly. It takes only about 10 minutes for the medication to work, and the resulting erection usually lasts at least 30 minutes. The cost is about $100 for as many as 15 to 20 injections, and most insurance companies will cover the expense.

Injections must be limited to three times a week to prevent the risk of injuring or scarring the penis. Also, in a small number of cases, injections can cause a condition called priapism, in which the erection continues for a long but unhealthy period of time. Because the blood in the penis is trapped, it thickens due to loss of oxygen, which can damage the penile tissue. If priapism occurs, placing a towel-covered ice pack over the penis usually

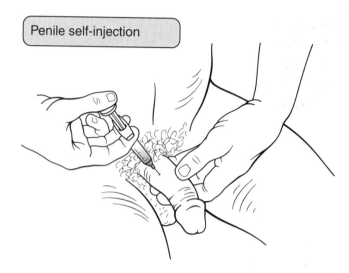

Penile self-injection

FIGURE Q-3.—In Pharmacologic Therapy (penile self-injection), the patient injects a drug into the side of his penis, which causes blood to flow into the organ, producing a strong erection.

solves the problem. If, despite the ice pack, the erection does not go away, a doctor should be called immediately because this is considered an emergency.

The proper dosage for injection is determined by trial and error. Some men require a small dosage while others require a large amount. It is essential for the man and his doctor to determine the proper dosage before self-injection can begin. If the man's partner wants to give the injection this is also encouraged, because it can actually be stimulating for both parties to incorporate this into foreplay.

A gel that can be rubbed on the penis for the treatment of impotence may soon gain FDA approval. This gel, made by MacroChem, contains the same active ingredient used in penile injection therapy.

Testosterone Injections. While these have received some attention, they should not be given to treat erectile problems after prostate surgery because testosterone could encourage the growth of any prostate cancer cells that could be left in the body.

Vacuum Constriction Devices. These devices consist of a large plastic tube, a pump, lubrication, and a rubber band or elastic ring. The tube is placed over the lubricated penis and the pump is used to create a vacuum, or suction, inside the tube, which causes blood to flow into the penis and a strong erection to result. The ring or rubber band is then taken off the tube and placed around the bottom of the penis to keep the blood inside the organ so that the erection can be maintained. The erection ends when the band or ring is removed (up to 30 minutes later). This device can work for men with nerve damage because it manually brings blood into the penis. And, as long as this device is not used for more than 30 minutes at a time, it can be used several times a week.

However, there are potential drawbacks to these devices. Some men feel that the ring or elastic band is uncomfortable and that the penis feels colder because there is no blood circulation. Others complain that it looks unnatural to wear the ring or use the device. Regardless, the devices are effective and the companies that make them usually have videos and sales representatives who can answer any questions and handle any concerns. A good device can cost up to $500, but Medicare and many insurance companies will cover some of the cost. Most also come with a trial period and a money-back guarantee. A doctor's prescription is needed for these devices.

Penile Implants (*prostheses*). Implants are another popular solution for erectile problems. While they do not allow the head of the penis to swell as well as it would naturally, they are still effective in producing an erection.

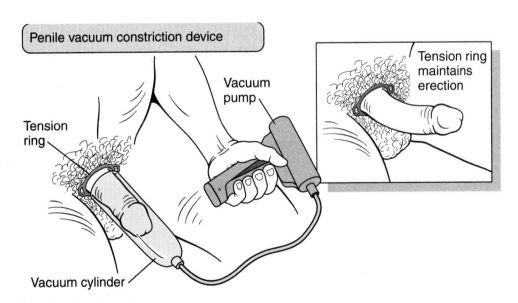

FIGURE Q-4—The Vacuum Constriction Device involves the use of vaccum, or suction, to draw blood into the penis and produce an erection. Once the penis is erect, a ring or rubber band is placed round the base of the penis to keep the blood inside the organ. The erection lasts as long as the band is in place.

There are four types of penile implants:

▶ **The Malleable, or Bendable, Implant.** This is also called the semi-rigid penile prosthesis. It is the easiest device to implant and the least likely to malfunction. It is a collection of wires within a silicone covering. Once implanted, the penis stays erect constantly with this device, which is manually adjusted.

▶ **The Mechanical Implant.** This device is a spring-loaded steel cable encased in a series of interlocking plastic blocks. It is very similar to the malleable implant, except the penis does not become erect until the device is manually locked in place. In addition, it is easier to bend—a plus for people who are not as strong with their hands, such as those with arthritis.

▶ **Inflatable Implant without Pump.** When the tip of this device is squeezed in the glans (head) of the penis it causes fluid within the implant to shift around and the penis then becomes hard. When the implant is bent and a release valve is used, the erection subsides.

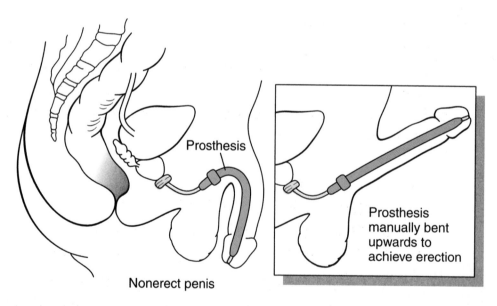

FIGURE Q-5.—The malleable Penile Implant consists of a collection of wires within a silicone covering. Once surgically implanted, the penis stays erect constantly and can be manually adjusted upward or downward.

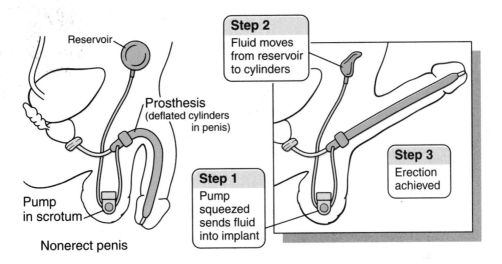

FIGURE Q-6.—The Inflatable Penile Implant with pump, provides the most natural erection of any of the devices, allowing the penis to be flaccid (limp) as well as erect. When an erection is desired, a pump implanted into the scrotum is squeezed; this sends fluid into the implant, which produces an erection.

▶ **Inflatable Implant with Pump.** This implant provides the most natural erection of any of the devices. In addition to an implant, a pump is placed into the scrotum between the testicles. When the pump is squeezed, it allows fluid to flow into the implant, thus causing an erection. Since this is a more complicated device, there is the slight chance of a complication that may require additional surgery.

All of the implants are inserted into the penis through either an incision directly into the penis or in the lower abdominal wall. Most of these procedures can be done on an outpatient basis. One must wait about four to six weeks after the surgery before resuming sexual activity. This time allows the area to heal. Implants are meant to be permanent; if removed, erection will be impossible by any other means.

Complications of implants can include infection, which requires antibiotic therapy and/or removal of the device; erosion, in which the implant can extend through the urethra or even the side of the penis; torque, in which the wires of the implant can twist on each other causing the penis to twist; pain, which can be treated with medication; and general malfunction or the need for replacement.

Depending on the implant, the price can range from a few thousand dollars to $20,000 for the device and the operation to implant it. The more technical the implant, the higher the price. Many insurance companies cover the cost of these devices.

Section

4

Hormonal Therapy for Prostate Cancer

HORMONE THERAPY

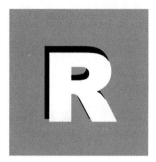

HORMONE THERAPY IS OFTEN USED TO CONTROL THE CANCER, WHEN PROSTATE CANCER IS THOUGHT TO BE OUTSIDE THE PROSTATE, OR WHEN IT IS KNOWN TO HAVE SPREAD TO OTHER ORGANS.

HORMONES ARE SUBSTANCES PRODUCED BY ONE PART OF THE BODY THAT TRAVEL IN THE BLOODSTREAM TO AFFECT OTHER PARTS OF THE BODY. IN MEN, THE PRIMARY HORMONE IS TESTOSTERONE, WHICH PLAYS A ROLE IN EVERYTHING FROM THE DEPTH OF VOICE TO THE GROWTH OR LOSS OF HAIR.

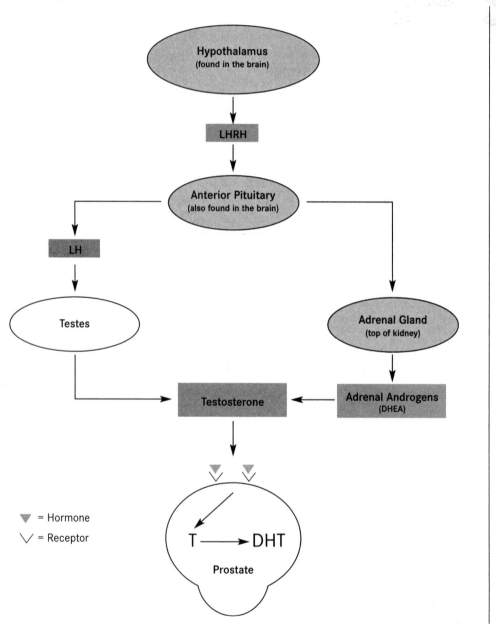

FIGURE R-1.—How testosterone is made and what happens when it gets into the prostate.

▶ Testosterone

There is a structure in the brain called the hypothalamus that makes luteinizing hormone-releasing hormone (LHRH). LHRH travels from the hypothalamus to the anterior pituitary, which is also in the brain, to create luteinizing hormone (LH), which travels to the testicles, where it causes cells to make testosterone (a hormone).

Many prostate cancer cells need testosterone to grow. Testosterone belongs to a class of hormones called "androgens." Cancer cells that grow faster and do more damage when hormones are present are called "hormone-sensitive cancer cells." Cancer cells that grow at a pace that is unaffected by hormones are called "hormone-insensitive cancer cells." Prostate cancer consists of both types of cells, and every man's ratio of sensitive to insensitive cells is different. The more hormone-sensitive cells there are, the better the response to hormone therapy. The more hormone-insensitive cells there are, the less successful the results will be from hormone therapy.

Hormonal therapy is essentially the elimination of testosterone.

This can be done in a number of ways:

▶ The testicles can be removed.

▶ An LHRH injection can be given.

▶ An antiandrogen pill can be taken.

▶ An antiandrogen pill can be taken after the testicles have been removed.

▶ An LHRH injection can be given along with an antiandrogen pill (or the pill can be given later).

One approach to stop the production of testosterone is to remove the testicles, a procedure known as "bilateral orchiectomy" or "surgical castration." When the testicles are removed, the production of testosterone stops almost immediately—or at least most of it does. About 5% to 10% of the body's testosterone is actually made in the adrenal glands, located on the top of the kidneys.

Equally effective as an orchiectomy is to give LHRH analog injections. The LHRH analogs cause the body to "think" that there is too much LHRH in the system, and to become desensitized to the hormone. Thus, the body begins to ignore LHRH; the anterior pituitary no longer recognizes it, and so it stops releasing LH, which in turn causes the testicles to stop making testosterone. (When a course of LHRH injections begins, there is actually a large initial increase in testosterone production, but after a few days, desensitization takes effect and the testosterone production drops.) Injections of LHRH can be given every month, every three months, every four months, or yearly depending on the type of medicine. Two of the most commonly used LHRHa injections are the Lupron® injection, which is usually given in the buttocks or hip, and the Zoladex® injection, which is usually injected in the abdomen. These injections work about the same. Viadur® is an LHRH analog that is given as an implant, usually in the arm, through a small surgical incision. It lasts for one year.

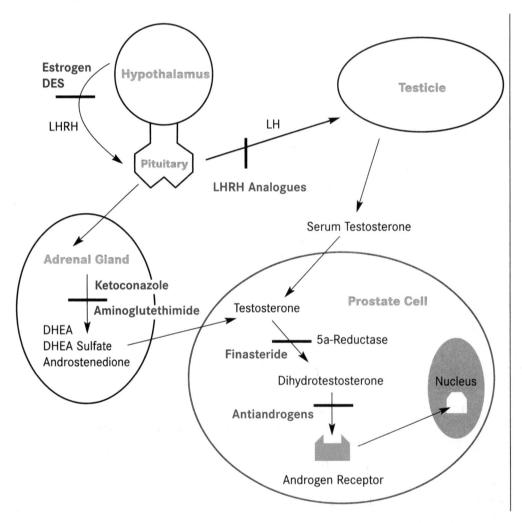

FIGURE R-2.—Summary of first and potential second-line therapies for prostate cancer.

► Hormonal Therapy

In general, hormonal therapy induces a remission in 80% to 90% of men with advanced prostate cancer. In general, it holds the cancer in check for an average of two to three years. In some patients, the cancer is put into remission for even longer. The majority of patients gradually develop a recurrence of their cancer which is then termed "androgen independent" or "hormone refractory".

Hormonal ablation can be performed in a variety of ways.

Common Names for Hormonal Ablation

Hormonal ablation can be performed in a variety of ways. It has a variety of names.

▶ Adjuvant hormonal therapy or treatment (given before, during, or after a precedure)
▶ Adjuvant and neoadjuvant therapy or treatment (given before, during or after a procedure)
▶ Androgen blockade
▶ Androgen deprivation
▶ Antiandrogen treatment
▶ Bilateral orchiectomy (also known as medical castration)
▶ Combined hormonal treatment
▶ Double-agent androgen deprivation
▶ Hormonal therapy and hormonal treatment (These terms are commonly used, but are somewhat inaccurate, because doctors are not providing hormones, they are eliminating them.)
▶ LHRH treatment
▶ Maximal androgen blockade (MAB)
▶ Monotherapy
▶ Neoadjuvant Hormonal therapy or treatment (given before a certain procedure)
▶ Single agent androgen deprivation

It has a variety of names:

▶ Adjuvant hormonal therapy or treatment (given after another procedure)

▶ Adjuvant and neoadjuvant therapy or treatment (given before, during, or after a procedure)

▶ Androgen ablation

▶ Androgen blockade

▶ Androgen deprivation

▶ Antiandrogen treatment

▶ Bilateral orchiectomy (also known as medical castration)

▶ Combined hormonal treatment

▶ Double-agent androgen deprivation

▶ Hormonal therapy and hormonal treatment (These terms are commonly used, but are somewhat inaccurate, because doctors are not providing hormones, they are eliminating them.)

▶ LHRH treatment

▶ Maximal androgen blockade (MAB)

▶ Monotherapy

▶ Neoadjuvant Hormonal therapy or treatment (given before a certain procedure)

▶ Single agent androgen deprivation

▶ Why and When Should Hormone Therapy Begin?

Hormonal ablation is used to treat men with prostate cancer at all stages of the disease, but it is usually given to those with either locally-advanced, regionally-advanced, or metastatic cancer. Hormonal ablation is not used as a cure for prostate cancer. There are some cases in which men show no signs of cancer after hormonal ablation, but it is most often used to control the disease and provide relief from symptoms.

THE STANDARD METHODS OF HORMONAL THERAPY

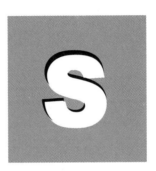

SURGICAL CASTRATION
OR
"BILATERAL ORCHIECTOMY"

The word "bilateral" refers to "both" (in this case both testicles), the prefix "orchi" means "testicles," and the suffix "ectomy" means "the removal of." Basically, it is the medical terminology for castration. Only the testicles themselves are removed during the procedure, not the scrotum. The spermatic cord is also left, which helps retain the natural appearance of the scrotum. To ensure an even more natural look, an artificial testicular implant can be placed in the scrotum during the surgery.

After surgery, the production of testosterone stops almost immediately—or at least most of it does. About 5% to 10% of the body's testosterone is actually produced in the adrenal glands, located on the top of the kidneys. Surgical castration is one of the original treatments for advanced prostate cancer since it was a known treatment long before the

175

LHRH agonists were developed. It is an inexpensive and effective form of hormonal therapy; however, it does have drawbacks. First, it may be psychologically hard for a man to lose his testicles. Second, surgical castration removes the option of newer potential therapies such as intermittent androgen blockade, where men are cycled on and off LHRH therapy. On the positive side, men do not have to be bothered by regular injections of the LHRH agonists and the treatment works equally well as the injection therapies.

The advantages of bilateral orchiectomy:

▶ It is easy and inexpensive (as compared with the other treatment options for advanced prostate cancer).

▶ It can be done on an outpatient basis.

▶ Even though the testicles are removed, the scrotum remains, which maintains a normal appearance.

▶ It is very effective in reducing the amount of testosterone in the body.

▶ Its impact is immediate: almost all of the body's testosterone is gone within hours after the surgery, and there is no chance of it returning because its main production source has been eliminated.

▶ Although it is a permanent procedure that cannot be reversed, it can increase the quality and quantity of life.

The disadvantages of bilateral orchiectomy:

▶ It causes a decreased sex drive, or libido, in most men.

▶ It causes erectile dysfunction (the decreased ability to have an erection) or impotence in most men.

▶ It is unable to eliminate the small amount (5% to 10%) of testosterone produced by the adrenal glands that continues to circulate in the body.

▶ It causes hot flashes, similar to those that women get during menopause, in about half of those who undergo the procedure. However, there are a number of medications that can treat these symptoms, such as estrogen, Megace®, Provera®, and clonidine.

▶ It causes slight breast enlargement (also called gynecomastia) and nipple tenderness or sensitivity in about half of those who have the surgery.

▶ It causes weight gain around the midsection (between 10 and 15 pounds).

▶ It is not reversible.

▶ Another possible anxiety is psychological; potentially feeling a loss of manhood.

▶ LHRH Agonists

There are some very good nonsurgical alternatives to bilateral orchiectomy. The first is a form of single-agent hormonal therapy that uses a class of drugs called "LHRH agonists." The best candidates for LHRH agonists are men with locally-advanced prostate cancer (stages C, T3 or T4) or cancer that has spread to other parts of the body (stages D, T3, T4, N+ or M+).

Some of the commonly prescribed LHRH agonists include leuprolide acetate (Lupron®), made by Abbott Laboratories; and goserelin acetate (Zoladex®), made by AstraZeneca Pharmaceuticals. The Lupron® injection, is usually given in the buttocks, and the Zoladex® injection, is usually injected in the abdomen. These injections only take seconds, and they both work about the same. These injections must be taken throughout life unless the man decides to have a bilateral orchiectomy.

The first time an LHRH agonist is injected, it temporarily increases testosterone production for 7 to 10 days. This brief surge can cause a condition called "tumor flare" in about 10% to 30% of men, in which symptoms temporarily become worse. However, an antiandrogen medication can be given at the same time to prevent the testosterone spike. After the first week to 10 days, the agonist starts working to shut off testosterone. Therefore, the eventual effect is similar to a bilateral orchiectomy in that the body's testosterone level drops to near zero. A new medication, Abarelix®, is being developed as an LHRH antagonist. This drug will not require antiandrogens to block the "flare response."

LHRH injections can be given every month, every three months, or every four months. The longer-lasting injections are certainly more convenient, but some health professionals feel that such long intervals tend to limit personal interaction between the individual and his doctor.

The advantages of LHRH agonists:

▶ They are as effective as testicle-removal surgery in decreasing testosterone levels to near zero.

▶ They are as effective as surgery in increasing the quality and quantity of life.

▶ Testicle-removal surgery can still be an option later on.

The disadvantages of LHRH agonists:

▶ They cause decreased libido, or sex drive, in most men.

▶ They cause erectile dysfunction or impotence in most men.

▶ They may require the additional use of an antiandrogen medication at the beginning of treatment to prevent tumor flare.

▶ They cause hot flashes similar to those experienced by women during menopause. However, there are a number of medications that can treat this uncomfortable symptom.

▶ They cause slight breast enlargement and nipple tenderness or sensitivity in about half of the men who take them. However, this can be prevented with several low-dosage radiation treatments to the breast (also can be done with bilateral orchiectomy patients).

▶ They cause weight gain around the midsection (between 10 and 15 pounds) in most men.

▶ They require regular trips to the doctor for injections for the rest of the man's life.

▶ They can cause the testicles to decrease in size.

▶ The injections are expensive, about $4,000 – $6,000 a year, but are covered by most health insurances.

LHRH agonists reduce the levels of testosterone in the blood, usually causing a reduction in the tumor and producing a decrease in PSA. The PSA decreases in over 90% of men and will often become undetectable.

▶ Combined Hormonal Therapy

In single-agent hormonal therapy, one drug or one procedure causes a dramatic decrease in a testosterone. However, research has shown that up to 10% of the total hormone levels within the prostate can come from the adrenal glands. Combination androgen-deprivation therapy [also called combined hormonal therapy (CHT); maximal androgen blockade (MAB); complete androgen blockade (CAB); or total androgen blockade (TAB)] pairs an LHRH agonist or bilateral orchiectomy with an antiandrogen drug to block this additional source of testosterone from stimulating the prostate cancer cells to grow.

Inside the body, circulating testosterone enters prostate cancer cells and binds to "androgen receptors." Androgen receptors are then activated and allow the cells to grow. The antiandrogen drugs bicalutamide, flutamide, and nilutamide block, in part, circulating testosterone from binding to the androgen receptors. These drugs are not approved for use as single agents and, if used, are administered in combination with the LHRH agonists. The effectiveness of high-dose antiandrogens as a single agent is currently being evaluated.

Although many doctors are satisfied with the results of medical or surgical castration, some believe that an antiandrogen should also be given to eliminate the testosterone and other androgens produced by the adrenal glands. Proponents of this combined approach think that CHT may:

▶ Provide a better initial response by preventing tumor flare.

▶ Delay the development of more hormone-insensitive prostate cancer cells.

▶ Slow the progression of prostate cancer.

▶ Increase survival.

None of these things have been proven. Monotherapy (single drug therapy with Lupron® or Zolodex®) and CAB can both be considered standards of care for men with metastatic disease. Some doctors use monotherapy, and others use complete androgen blockade. It is a matter of preference. What is known is that an antiandrogen should initially be used in combination with an LHRH agonist to prevent a flare response if men have known metastatic disease. This is only a temporary problem and the antiandrogen can be stopped after the first month if the man is going to continue on monotherapy.

The antiandrogens include bicalutamide, flutamide, nilutamide, and cyproterone acetate.

Bicalutamide (trade name Casodex®)

This is a commonly used antiandrogen that is taken once per day. It is difficult to determine the exact side-effects of this medicine because it is given with the LHRH analogs. However, reported side effects include:

▶ Hot flashes (in 40% of men)

- Nausea (in 10% of men)
- Nipple tenderness (in 5% of men)
- Itching (in 5% of men)
- Breast enlargement, or "gynecomastia" (in 5% of men)
- Changes in blood test parameters which reflect liver function (less than 5% of men)

Flutamide (trade name Eulexin®)

Another commonly used antiandrogens is flutamide. It is an oral drug that is given two to three times a day. Some of its side effects are:

- Hot flashes (in approximately 60% of men)
- Diarrhea (in approximately 10% of men)
- Breast enlargement, or "gynecomastia" (in approximately 10% of men)
- Liver problems (in approximately 5% to 10% of men)

Nilutamide (trade name Nilandron®)

Nilutamide is another antiandrogen. Its side effects include:

- Hot flashes (in 25% to 30% of men)
- Impaired vision in the dark (in 10% to 15% of men)
- Nausea (in 10% of men)
- Constipation (in 5% to 10% of men)
- Dizziness (in 5% to 10% of men)
- Lung inflammation, or pneumonitis (in 1% to 5% of men)

Men who are on combined androgen blockade are taken off their antiandrogen medicine if their cancer begins to grow and their PSA level increases. This is because that in some men, the cancer has changed or mutated, and the antiandrogens may actually encourage the cancer to grow. This is called the "anti - androgen withdrawal syndrome" and is found with all of the antiandrogens. Studies have demonstrated that approximately 25%

of men will have their PSA decrease when the antiandrogen is stopped. This PSA decrease lasts approximately 4 to 6 months in most patients.

Men who are on monotherapy are often started on an antiandrogen to see if combined androgen blockade will control their cancer. This works in about 10% of men.

Cyproterone Acetate (CPA) ~ (also called) Androcur®

Cyproterone acetate (CPA) is a steroidal, progestational antiandrogen that blocks the androgen-receptor interaction and reduces testosterone through a weak anti-gonadotropic action. It is commonly used in Canada as monotherapy or as an agent to prevent disease flare during initiation of LHRH agonist therapy. CPA can also suppress hot flashes in response to androgen deprivation treatment with LHRH agonists or bilateral orchiectomy. Although it is generally well tolerated, CPA is also associated with a high rate of breast enlargement/tenderness and/or a small number of cardiovascular complications, and is not available in the United States but doctors do prescribe it in Europe, Canada, and other parts of the world.

▶ Triple Androgen Blockade

Another therapy that a few physicians have started to use is called triple androgen blockade. In this therapy, Finasteride (Proscar®) is added to CAB. Finasteride is the drug that blocks the conversion of testosterone to its more active breakdown product, dihydrotestosterone. Currently, there is no clear evidence that this is an effective treatment for hormone-sensitive prostate cancer.

HORMONAL THERAPY IN CONJUNCTION WITH LOCAL THERAPY

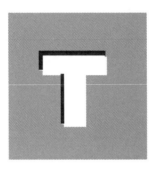

WHEN IS HORMONAL ABLATION USED?

HORMONAL ABLATION IS SOMETIMES USED BY ITSELF FOR MEN WHO HAVE UNDERGONE WATCHFUL WAITING; HOWEVER, ITS USE FOR MEN WITH LOCALLY-ADVANCED (OR SUSPECTED TO BE LOCALLY-ADVANCED) CANCER IS OCCURRING MORE AND MORE. THAT IS, IT CAN BE GIVEN IN THE NEOADJUVANT SETTING (PRIOR TO THE START OF TREATMENT), THE CONCURRENT SETTING (DURING TREATMENT), AND THE ADJUVANT SETTING (AFTER TREATMENT).

▶ Hormonal Ablation and Surgery

Neoadjuvant Therapy

Hormonal ablation is sometimes given prior to surgery (neoadjuvant therapy) to try to reduce the size of the cancer in order to make it easier to remove, or in order to stop it from growing beyond the immediate area of the prostate. It is most likely to be recommended for men who have a high risk of having positive surgical margins—those with stage T2b or higher disease, PSA levels greater than 10 – 20 ng/ml, and a high Gleason score.

In general, studies have found a consistent decrease in prostate size and PSA with neoadjuvant therapy and surgery. Prostate size was reduced anywhere from 40% to 90%, and in virtually all the studies, 100% of the men had a decrease in PSA. In addition, most trials have shown a significantly lower number of positive surgical margins—about a 10% to 30% decrease—in patients having neoadjuvant therapy versus those having only surgery.

There are, of course, drawbacks to this approach. Men are on hormonal therapy from between three and eight months prior to surgery. Some experts believe that this may give the hormone resistant cells that may be present in the cancer more time to grow. In addition, some reports suggest that it can actually make surgery more difficult, because the prostate experiences a type of scarring or fibrosis reaction that makes it difficult to identify the prostate margins and to cleanly cut the prostate out. In addition, the evidence is not clear at this time whether or not hormones given before surgery are effective in decreasing the chance of the cancer recurring.

Adjuvant Therapy

It is unclear if hormone therapy should be used after prostatectomy. Some studies have suggested that men with disease outside the prostate at the time of surgery (pT3b) (locally-advanced) may benefit from undergoing hormone therapy immediately. In one analysis by the Mayo Clinic, adjuvant therapy was associated with a significant improvement in biochemical progression-free survival (67% versus 23% at 10 years), systemic progression-free survival (90% versus 78%), and cause-specific survival (95% versus 87%).

The Eastern Cooperative Oncology Group (ECOG) followed 98 men with positive lymph nodes at the time of surgery. Half of the men received immediate hormonal therapy

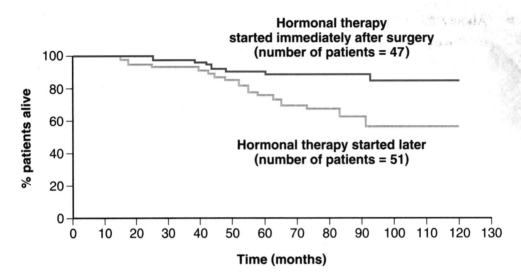

FIGURE T-1.—Overall survival in men receiving prostatectomy plus adjuvant hormonal therapy (bilateral orchiectomy or goserelin) compared with prostatectomy and deferred hormonal treatment.

(with either goserelin or bilateral orchiectomy) and the other half were treated with hormone therapy at the time of cancer progression. The men treated with hormone therapy immediately after surgery seemed to do better and live longer than the men who had deferred treatment.

Hormonal Ablation and Radiation Therapy

Hormonal ablation is sometimes used with radiation therapy because it may reduce the number of cells that need to be destroyed by radiation, and it may make cancer cells more vulnerable.

Concurrent and Adjuvant Therapy in Radiation Therapy Patients

In 1998, a study showed that men with T3 and T4 prostate cancer may keep cancer away longer and live longer if they are given hormonal ablation as soon as radiation therapy is started, and then for three years after treatment. In this study:

- About 80% of the men receiving combined treatment were alive five years after treatment, versus a little more than 60% of the men receiving only radiation.
- Of the patients who were alive after five years, 85% had no signs of disease, versus 48% of those who received radiation alone.

This appears to be great news for men with locally-advanced prostate cancer, but more research is still needed. Also, there are some things to remember when considering these results. For example:

- The men in the study were either given radiation therapy or radiation therapy with hormonal ablation. There were no men in the study who received hormonal ablation alone. It could be that men would do just as well on hormonal ablation with no other treatment.
- The study only followed men for about four years—the rest of the data was based on estimates.
- Men who were given the combined treatment experienced more incontinence (about 30% versus about 15%), and naturally experienced more hormonal ablation-related side effects such as hot flashes (in about 60% of the men).

Overall, there are still a lot of unknowns with hormonal ablation used in conjunction with radiation therapy. But it does seem to be a promising option, so it worth discussing with the doctor. It is now generally accepted that men with prostate cancer that is thought to be at high risk of recurring should be treated with radiation therapy plus 2 – 3 years of hormonal therapy.

High Risk Prostate Cancers

- T2 cancer, any PSA, Gleason 8–10
- T2 cancer, PSA >20 ng/mL, Gleason 7
- T3 cancer, any PSA or Gleason score

NEW APPROACHES FOR HORMONAL THERAPY

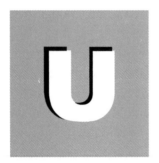

▶ **Immediate versus Delayed Hormone Therapy:**
  The Case of the Man with the Rising PSA

It is now becoming increasingly common that the only symptom in a man with advanced disease is a rising PSA level. (This is most frequently seen in someone who was treated for localized disease and whose bone scan and CT scan are still negative.) Alternatively, hormonal therapy may have cleared previously seen prostate cancer from bone scans or CT scans.

One area that is still being explored is the timing of treatment for advanced prostate cancer. That is, is it best to give hormonal ablation immediately after diagnosis, or to wait until the individual actually shows symptoms of the disease?

When men hear this they usually ask: "Why would I want to delay treatment?" The argument for delaying is that if a man has no symptoms of advanced disease, hormonal treatment will produce significant side effects at a time when they would otherwise feel good.

The argument against delayed treatment is more obvious. A rising PSA level means that the prostate cancer will eventually surface somewhere (most likely in the bones) and even if immediate treatment does not lead to better survival rates, delaying might increase the likelihood of problems with the bladder, urination, kidneys, and bones (for example, spinal cord compression).

Unfortunately, for men with PSA-only disease, experts do not know what the best answer is. Some believe treatment should begin right away, others wait until the PSA level reaches a specific number (10, 20, 50....), and still others favor waiting until there is either clinical or scan evidence of disease. Each situation is different and the matter should be discussed with the doctor.

▶ Immediate versus Delayed Hormone Therapy: The Case of Clinically Evident or Scan-positive Disease

This situation of when to treat appears to be clearer. The results from a large study started in 1985 indicate that progression of the prostate cancer is more likely to be slowed by immediate treatment. In this study, men with M0 disease and delayed treatment developed metastatic cancer faster, bone pain occurred earlier, and overall progression or advancement of disease was faster. Also, more of these men needed TURPs (30% of delayed-treatment men vs. 14% of immediate-treatment men). However, the authors of the study could not make an absolute recommendation applicable to all men with prostate cancer. The study is still going on, and more will be known in a few years. However, there is good evidence now to start hormonal therapy early in this situation. Ultimately, both the man and his doctor should be armed with as much information as possible concerning ongoing studies in this area. This will make the treatment decision-making process much easier.

▶ Intermittent Androgen Blockade (IAB)

Some doctors believe that hormone therapy may at times encourage the growth of both hormone-insensitive and aggressive prostate cancer cells. Based on laboratory studies that support this idea and the knowledge that hormonal therapy has side effects, a study was done that demonstrated that men on intermittent androgen blockade (IAB) therapy had a similar survival and an increased quality of life as compared to men on continuous hormonal therapy. To really know if this type of therapy is better, a study that directly compares the two therapies needs to be completed. While one is currently being conducted, the results will not be known for several years. Therefore, intermittent therapy is still considered experimental.

Although there are no absolute guidelines, intermittent therapy is usually administered by starting a man on CAB for approximately 6 to 8 months, until the PSA is undetectable. The man is then taken off CAB and his testosterone is allowed to rise. This allows the hormone-sensitive cells to start to grow. This will, of course, allow the PSA to start to rise. When the PSA reaches a point decided on by the doctor, the CAB is restarted and the cycle continues. Although it is not known if this therapy increases survival, it does appear to increase quality of life, and doctors are using this treatment more and more. In early studies, men reported a better quality of life during their off periods. One study demonstrated that while off treatment, 42% of men noted an improvement in energy; hot flushes disappeared in 60% and decreased in 33%; libido increased in 75%; and erections improved in 62%. Retrospective comparison of survival in men who underwent IAB was similar to those treated with continuous therapy. Of note, approximately 20% to 25% of men who undergo androgen ablation for 6 to 12 months do not recover their gonadal function and do not experience a rise in testosterone and relief of side effects when androgen blockade is stopped.

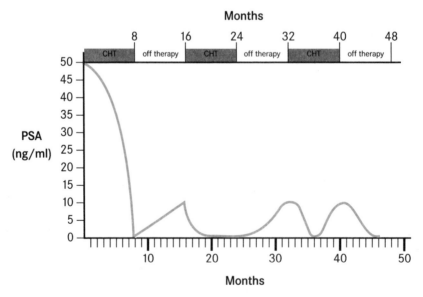

FIGURE U-1.—Intermittent Hormonal Therapy.

▶ Sequential Androgen Blockade (SAB)

Combining a nonsteroidal antiandrogen (flutamide, bicalutamide, nilutamide) with finasteride blocks the conversion of testosterone to its active metabolite dihydrotestosterone, and also prevents testosterone and dihydrotestosterone from binding to the androgen receptor. This approach, often termed sequential androgen blockade (SAB), results in androgen deprivation at the cellular level, but leaves circulating testosterone levels intact. In early trials, this therapy has resulted in a decrease in PSA level in the majority of men while maintaining their sexual potency. This form of treatment has not been tested against traditional androgen deprivation in a head – to – head trial, and its impact on survival remains unknown. While initially used mainly in men with advanced disease who wished to maintain potency, it is now being used in the experimental setting to treat men with bio-chemical failure following primary therapy (PSA-only disease). This type of treatment remains unproven and its impact is uncertain. At least one study, however, has demon-strated that approximately 80% of men treated with SAB respond to androgen depriva-tion therapy when their PSA level starts to rise. This suggests that SAB may become a first-line treatment of choice in the future for men with advanced prostate cancer.

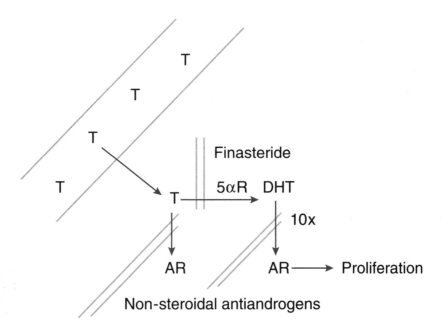

FIGURE U-2.—Sequential Androgen Blockade.

SIDE EFFECTS
OF HORMONAL THERAPY
AND THEIR
TREATMENT

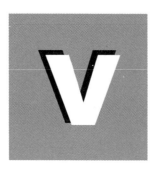

Hormonal therapy can generate a number of side effects, most of them are related to the decrease in male hormone levels. These side effects include:

- ▶ Anemia (10-20% of men)
- ▶ Bone density loss (almost all men to some degree)
- ▶ Cognitive function loss (this is still being studied)
- ▶ Depression (10-50% of men)

▶ Fatigue (the majority of men)

▶ High-density lipoprotein level decrease (10–30% of men)

▶ Hot flashes (about 50–80% of men)

▶ Impotence (inability to have an erection) (almost all men)

▶ Loss of libido or sex drive (almost all men)

▶ Muscle atrophy (almost all men to some degree)

▶ Sweating (10% to 15% of men)

▶ Weight gain (especially around the midsection) (almost all men)

Initially, hormonal therapy was considered to be well tolerated. Loss of libido was often the only adverse side effect that was thought about. Several other side effects have now been noted. These include fatigue, weight gain, depression, osteopenia (bone density loss), anemia, muscle atrophy, gynecomastia, hot flashes, loss of cognitive function, and decrease in high-density lipoprotein. Severe symptoms may warrant consideration of changing therapy. For example, men with severe hot flashes from LHRH agonists or bilateral orchiectomy will often have symptom relief with the addition of estrogen or a progesterone agent. Other medications, such as venlafaxine, have also been shown to reduce the severity of hot flashes. The antiandrogens and cyproterone are associated with a rare but potentially fatal liver damage, and should be used with caution in men with pre-existing liver disease. Men on therapy should have their liver enzyme monitored with blood tests. Gynecomastia can often be lessened with a very short course of radiation therapy to the breasts, but only if initiated prior to hormonal therapy. For men who desire preservation of potency, high-dose antiandrogen therapy or a combination of finasteride and antiandrogen may be warranted as first-line treatment.

▶ Bone Density Loss

Once initiated, most men remain on hormonal therapy for years, if not the rest of their lives. Long-term treatment with androgen deprivation can lead to debilitating osteoporosis. Even in a study of intermittent androgen blockade, evaluation of bone mineral density in the lumbar spine and hip revealed osteopenia in 46% and osteoporosis in 20% of men. A similar study found that 50% of men on androgen blockade for at least 12 months had asymptomatic fractures in the bones of their spine. The precise incidence of clinically relevant fractures remains undefined.

The latest studies in elderly men with prostate cancer suggest that many have a deficiency of vitamin D and/or calcium and/or testosterone. However, taking daily supplements of calcium and vitamin D is not easy over a long period of time. In addition, the exact dose that men should take of these supplements is not exactly known. There has also been some concern that calcium may increase the risk of prostate cancer but the dosages have been very high in these studies.

Dietary/Lifestyle Supplement Recommendations for Men Concerned About Osteoporosis or those on Androgen Suppression Treatment for Prostate Cancer	
Complementary Therapy	**Dosage**
Elemental calcium (supplements)	At least 500–1000 mg daily
Vitamin D (supplements)	At least 700–800 IU daily
Dietary calcium	At least 500–700 mg daily
Dietary vitamin D	Several fish servings a week, and healthy fortified vitamin D foods and beverages
Dietary soy products	1–2 servings daily
Physical activity	Several times weekly
Weight bearing exercise	Several times weekly
Other	Do not smoke. Drink alcohol only in moderation, if at all. Moderate sun exposure helps the body produce vitamin D.

Bisphosphonates

Another way to prevent bone loss in men on hormonal therapy is through the use of diphosphonates (also called bisphosphonates). Bisphosphonates fight the breakdown of bone, and there are several clinical trials underway to see if these drugs are effective in blocking the breakdown of bone, preventing the spread of prostate cancer, and treating painful bone metastases. Commonly used bisphosphonates include: Alendronate, Risedronate, Ibandronate, Etidronate, Clodronate, Pamidronate, and Zoledronate.

The U.S. Food and Drug Administration has recently approved zoledronic acid, the newest intravenous bisphosphonate, for the treatment of skeletal events in men with documented metastatic disease (both androgen-dependent and androgen-independent). Zoledronic acid has been evaluated in a randomized, placebo-controlled trial of 422 men with androgen-independent (hormone refractory) prostate cancer. Significantly fewer men in the zoledronic acid group needed narcotic pain medicine or experienced pathologic fractures. The time elapse to vertebral (the bone of the back) fracture and pathologic fracture was significantly longer in the treatment group. Pain control at 3 months and 9 months was also significantly improved.

Researchers are not sure if men without evidence of cancer in the bones should be placed on a bisphosphonate drug. They should at least be offered calcium and vitamin D supplements if they have some bone loss. However, whether or not drugs for osteoporosis prevention are safe long term in men with prostate cancer without cancer having reached the bones is not known at this time. Of course, if someone has cancer in the bones, these drugs are a strong potential option.

▶ Depression

About 25% of the men who have prostate cancer experience significant depression. It is very important to report signs of depression to the doctor as depression makes it harder to treat cancer. Some common symptoms of depression are difficulty sleeping, lack of appetite, fatigue, loss of will to do any activity, and loss of enjoyment in any activities.

Tricyclic antidepressant drugs take 2 to 4 weeks to really work, and some of them may aggravate problems with urination. SSRI drugs usually work faster, and have fewer urinary side effects than the tricyclic drugs. Also, some over-the-counter products—like St. John's Wort or SAM-e—seem to help in cases of mild depression.

In addition to taking such medications, it might be useful to consult a therapist. This is also true for spouses, partners, and other family members who may be having emotional difficulties as a result of someone they care about having prostate cancer.

▶ Hot Flashes

There are many ways of potentially reducing hot flashes. However, some of the best are:

▶ 800 IU or 800 mg of vitamin E (400 IU in the morning and 400 IU in the evening). This is the only time higher doses of vitamin E are acceptable.

▶ Antidepressants (Effexor®, Paxil®, . . .), Megace®, and prescribed estrogens (DES).

▶ Eat at least 1 or 2 servings of soy products and 1 or 2 tablespoons of flaxseed daily. The plant estrogen in soy and flaxseed should help reduce hot flashes. Try mixing 1/3 to 1/2 cup of soy protein powder or 1 or 2 cups of soy milk in a favorite drink. Tofu and whole soybeans are also a great source of estrogen. Drink smoothies.

▶ Limit caffeine intake.

▶ Limit strenuous exercise.

▶ Avoid very warm temperatures. An excessively warm room may initiate hot flashes or make them worse.

Other supplements reported to reduce hot flashes for women may also help men. They are listed below. There is very little research regarding any of these products, including proper dosage. Generally, one or two capsules daily should be sufficient.

▶ Bioflavonoids

▶ Evening primrose oil

▶ Black cohosh

▶ Blue cohosh

▶ Chasteberry (*Vitex agnus castus*)

▶ Ginseng (Panax ginseng)

▶ Licorice (*Glycyrrhiza glabra*)—not the candy but the herb

▶ Wild yam (*Dioscorea villosa*)

▶ Curcumin

▶ Red Clover

▶ PC-SPES or other estrogenic supplements

▶ Acupuncture for Hot Flashes

A recent small study from Sweden demonstrated the ability of acupuncture to potentially reduce hot flashes that are a result of prostate cancer treatment. Seven men with advanced prostate cancer who received hormonal ablation treatment also received acupuncture treatment for 30 minutes twice weekly and then once a week for 12 weeks. Six of these men completed at least 10 weeks of the acupuncture treatment. All experienced about 70% fewer hot flashes. Nearly 3 months after the treatments were finished there was still a 50% decrease in the number of hot flashes. Although further research needs to be completed, currently acupuncture may be a viable option for the treatment of hot flashes due to prostate cancer treatment.

NOTES

NOTES

NOTES

Section

5

Beyond

Primary

Hormonal

Treatment

SECOND-LINE HORMONAL TREATMENTS

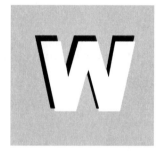

Hormonal ablation aims to kill cancer cells that depend on male hormones. Unfortunately, a tumor eventually becomes insensitive to hormonal ablation. Every tumor contains some hormone-sensitive (androgen dependent = AD) cells and some hormone-insensitive (androgen independent = AI) cells. After hormonal ablation, the AD cells die (and the PSA decreases), but the AI cells continue to grow. Eventually, the tumor contains only AI cells; it continues to grow, and the PSA rises despite the hormone ablation. At this point, the cancer is said to be "hormone refractory," or not responsive to the removal of hormones.

PSA and Advanced Disease

Since 1992, PSA has been used to measure the response of advanced prostate cancer to various treatments. Several studies and trials have shown a direct relationship between decreases in PSA and shrinkage of measurable prostate tumors as well as increased survival for patients who decreased their PSA by greater than 50% from their baseline value.

A special note on the use of PSA and advanced prostate cancer. In localized disease, we can use a PSA of 4 as an upper limit of normal to screen for cancer—but this is not the case with androgen-independent cancers. Each tumor creates a unique amount of PSA, which is relative to each individual. That means each patient has his own unique starting point, or baseline; a patient may have a small amount of cancer and a high PSA, or a large amount of cancer and a low PSA.

So remember: it is essentially meaningless to compare your PSA to that of another patient. There are patients who have a PSA of less than 10 who have many bone metastases and need narcotics to control their pain. Other patients with PSAs over 1,000 have no pain. There is no magic PSA number that correlates with symptoms or death! The important thing is whether your PSA number goes up or down, because that generally (but not always) correlates with whether your cancer is growing or shrinking.

Someone on hormonal ablation whose cancer continues to progress has the option of undergoing second-line hormonal treatment. There are several second-line hormonal therapy options that can be explored. These include:

▶   Adding antiandrogens if on monotherapy
▶   Taking away antiandrogens if on combined hormonal blockade
▶   Estrogens
▶   Ketoconazole
▶   Steroids
▶   High-dose antiandrogens
▶   PC-SPES or other estrogenic supplements

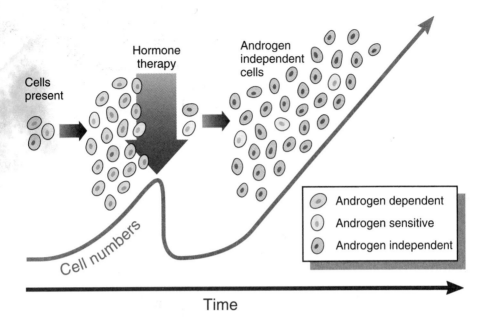

FIGURE W-1.—Hormone ablation to hormone refractory ranges.

▶ The Addition of an Antiandrogen

Occasionally, if a man on monotherapy experiences a rising PSA, his doctor will add an antiandrogen to his therapy. This slows the progression of the disease temporarily in approximately 10% of patients. Although this seems like a low number, it may be worth trying for someone with no symptoms.

Surgical Castration if Medical Castration Is not Working

A question commonly asked by men is whether they should have a surgical castration if the drugs are no longer working. If the testosterone result is at "castrate" level, then there is no need for surgery. This is the case almost all of the time.

A question commonly asked by men is whether they should have a surgical castration if the drugs are no longer working. If the testosterone result is at "castrate" level, then there is no need for surgery. This is the case almost all of the time.

▶ Antiandrogen Withdrawal Syndrome

Sometimes, the peripheral antiandrogens can actually begin to make the cancer grow after men take them for awhile. This appears to be due to the presence of altered or mutated androgen receptors that begin seeing the antiandrogen as an androgen. Therefore, when a rising PSA level is seen in men on CAB, the first step is to stop the antiandrogen (flutamide, bicalutamide, and nilutamide). This works to decrease the progression of the cancer in 10% to 30% of men for an average of 3 to 8 months. In addition, this syndrome can be observed with any hormonal treatment, so most doctors will look for it if someone has been taking any of the second-line hormone treatments.

▶ Estrogens

Estrogens go to the brain and decrease the amount of luteinizing hormone (LH) that is released. They may also be involved in the actual direct killing of prostate cancer cells. Initially there were cardiovascular problems associated with its use, but these can usually be minimized by using smaller dosages. A commonly used estrogen is diethylstilbestrol (DES).

One study found that DES as a second-line hormone given at 1 mg a day was effective in decreasing the PSA in 40% of men for an average of 8 months. DES appears to be a good option for men who have failed or are failing luteinizing hormone-releasing hormone (LHRH) therapy. Estrogens like DES are inexpensive ($5 – $15 dollars a month) and work as well as common hormonal ablation, but they fell out of favor years ago because they were associated with slightly more side effects. As a result, DES is difficult to find in the United States. Someone taking estrogen might also need to be on a blood-thinning drug (Coumadin® or Warfarin) or aspirin in order to reduce the chances of developing blood clots.

▶ Ketoconazole (trade name, Nizoral®)

Ketoconazole (trade name, Nizoral®), is a drug that blocks the production of testicular and adrenal androgens. It may also kill prostate cancer cells directly. The average dose is high—400 mg three times a day—and is associated with a large number of gastrointestinal problems. Objective responses of 15% and stable disease have been reported in about 30% of men. Stable disease means the cancer does not shrink or that the PSA level does not go down, but stays where it is for awhile. Ketoconazole is usually given with a steroid to replace the steroids that are no longer produced by the adrenal gland. More recently, this drug and hydrocortisone were used in men whose cancer progressed after experiencing flutamide (an antiandrogen) withdrawal. Out of 48 men:

▶ 45% – 50% had a greater than 80% PSA decrease for about 4 months.

▶ 60% – 65% had a greater than 50% PSA decrease for about 4 months.

▶ Glucocorticoids (Steroids)

Glucocorticoids prevent adrenal testosterone production. The three glucocorticoids most commonly used in the treatment of prostate cancer are:

▶ Prednisone®, which in one study was found to decrease pain in about 40% of men, and about 20% demonstrated a decrease in PSA for an average response of 4 months (but the range was 3 to 30 months).

▶ Hydrocortisone, which has led to a subjective response in up to 60% of men.

▶ Dexamethasone, which also has led to a subjective response in up to 60% of men.

▶ High-Dose Antiandrogens

In a study of 10 men with progressive metastatic prostate cancer who had failed CAB, and had received high-dose antiandrogens, 4 (or 40%) of the men felt better after therapy. Another study of high-dose antiandrogens looked at 52 men with advanced prostate cancer who showed disease progression following medical or surgical castration. There was no objective response seen, but almost a third of the men had stable disease and their self-pain score went down within three months after taking high-dose antiandrogens.

▶ PC-SPES and PC-Calm

PC-SPES, an herbal supplement, has been the subject of much controversy. The mechanism behind the effect of PC-SPES is not well understood. The toxicities and biochemical effects appear to be estrogenic. Analysis of the compound, however, did not yield any known estrogens. As PC-SPES is an herbal supplement, no standards exist for ensuring all pills have equal amounts of "active" extract. Recently, examination of some preparations of the supplement revealed the presence of a blood thinner and an anti-anxiety agent. It is also very expensive. At this time, PC-SPES has been taken off of the market. The fate of PC-SPES and its use in prostate cancer is unclear at this time. PC-Calm is a combination of several of the herbs in PC-SPES as well as some new ones. The identity of the components of PC-Calm is not readily available at this time. This supplement should not be taken without first contacting the doctor. It has the potential to interact with many prescription drugs.

In summary, there are several treatments that the doctor may want to discuss if first-line medical or surgical castration fails.

CHEMOTHERAPY

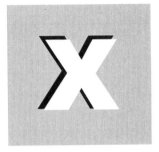

WHAT ARE THE STANDARD CHEMOTHERAPY OPTIONS AND WHEN SHOULD THEY BE USED?

RADIATION THERAPY AND SURGERY ARE MOST EFFECTIVE IN TREATING LOCALIZED PROSTATE CANCER, OR IN SIMPLY SLOWING ADVANCED CANCER. HORMONAL THERAPY IS MORE OFTEN USED FOR ADVANCED CANCER, BUT IT IS USEFUL FOR ONLY A LIMITED TIME, BECAUSE MEN BECOME "HORMONE-REFRACTORY," OR INSENSITIVE TO SUCH THERAPY, AFTER ABOUT TWO TO THREE YEARS, ON AVERAGE. AT THAT POINT, DOCTORS OFTEN TURN TO CHEMOTHERAPY TO FIGHT THE CANCER.

Chemotherapy refers to the use of drugs that attack and kill cancer cells. There are many different types of chemotherapy drugs that kill cancer cells in different ways. Some attach themselves to the DNA and do not allow it to copy itself. Others stop the cancer cells from dividing. All chemotherapy drugs work by killing cells that are dividing. Cancer cells grow faster than normal cells in the body and that is why chemotherapy works. It is also why people who take chemotherapy often lose their hair, because it also grows rapidly and the chemotherapy drugs kill the hair cells temporarily.

For many years, chemotherapeutic drugs for hormone refractory prostate cancer were used and analyzed as single agents given alone and in combination with other drugs, with poor results. In general, the average survival rate in these studies was something like six to nine months. Over the last five years, multiple new effective drugs and regimens have become available and the survival and quality of life of men with hormone-refractory disease is increasing. Results of chemotherapy can vary widely. It really comes down to looking at each individual and how he is going to be treated for his hormone-refractory prostate cancer.

At present, there are only a few standard approaches to treating men who are hormone-refractory. However, the National Comprehensive Cancer Network (NCCN), an organization of cancer centers around the country, has reviewed all of the studies that have been done recently on hormone-refractory disease and has set guidelines for care. These therapies are all new in the last five years and more are coming. Again, the drugs were chosen based on demonstrated anticancer activity and acceptable toxicity. The combinations include:

▶ Ketoconazole (Nizoral®) and Doxorubicin (Adriamycin®)

In one study, a combination of Ketoconazole (Nizoral®) and Doxorubicin (Adriamycin®) produced a PSA decrease of more than 50% in 55% of men. About 29% of the men developed complications such as acral erythema (redness of the hands and feet) and stomatitis (mouth sores). However, once Doxorubicin was stopped, the symptoms disappeared. When a symptom went away, the Doxorubicin was resumed and the symptoms did not return. The overall NCCN statistics for this combination are:

Continued Androgen Suppression

A controversial area in the treatment of androgen-independent prostate cancer has been whether a man who is going to take chemotherapy for hormone-refractory prostate cancer should stay on hormone therapy. In the past, most men with metastatic prostate cancer were treated with surgical castration either as first-line treatment or at the time of failure of hormone therapy via injections. Most men enrolling in clinical trials for androgen-independent disease still received some form of androgen ablation. With the widespread availability of medical forms of reversible hormone therapy using LHRH agonists (Lupron® or Zoladex®) and/or antiandrogens, the question of the role of continued hormone therapy in hormone-refractory disease has become important. A retrospective review of men enrolled in chemotherapy trials for androgen-independent disease tried to answer this question. It was concluded that continued hormone therapy was not a significant factor in survival. However, another review showed a modest survival advantage for men with continued hormone therapy. Also, many men feel more secure remaining on hormone therapy. At this time, it is the general consensus of oncologists (cancer specialists) to keep men on hormone therapy while new therapies are evaluated for hormone-refractory prostate cancer.

Response Rate:

The response rate tells you how many patients respond to a given treatment—usually this correlates with living longer.

▶ PSA response in 55% of men (doctors define a PSA response as a >50% decrease in PSA from baseline that is held for at least 4 weeks).

▶ Soft tissue response in 60% of men (a soft tissue response is measured in two ways:

 ▶ a partial response (PR) is a 50% decrease in the size of a measurable mass (usually a lymph node on a CT scan), or

 ▶ a complete response (CR), which is complete disappearance of the lesion).

Side Effects:

▶ A few men (2) died suddenly from treatment.
▶ Stomatitis and acral erythema: 30% of men.
▶ Serious anal mucositis in 13% of men (sloughing of the inner lining of the lower gastrointestinal tract, which causes very painful bowel movements, diarrhea, and bleeding temporarily).

▶ Vinblastine (Velban®) and Estramustine (Emyct®)

The combination of Vinblastine and Estramustine seems to enhance tumor killing in preclinical models of prostate cancer. In clinical trials, PSA decreases of more than 50% were found in 54% to 61% of the men. This therapy was well tolerated—meaning it produced relatively few side effects. One trial showed that men who experienced a greater than 50% decline in PSA had significantly increased overall and progression-free survival. The overall NCCN statistics for this combination are:

Response Rate:

▶ PSA response in 55% to 60% of men.
▶ Soft tissue response in 15% to 40% of men.

Side Effects:

▶ Nausea in 20% of men.
▶ Leukopenia (decrease in white blood cells) in 12% of men.
▶ Constipation in 20% of men.
▶ Transient neuropathy in 12% of men (neuropathy is a condition that causes numbness and tingling in the hands and feet).

▶ Etoposide (VePesid®) and Estramustine

In laboratory tests, the combination of Etoposide and Estramustine has been shown to kill cancer cells and impair the replication of DNA by the cancer cell. In a clinical trial, a PSA decrease of greater than 50% was demonstrated in 55% of men. Estramustine caused significant nausea in about 30% of men. Other trials that used a lower dose of Estramustine showed a PSA decrease of greater than 50% in about 40% of the men, with less nausea. It is advisable to take Estramustine with food. Calcium-rich products such as milk, yogurt, ice cream, antacids containing calcium, should be avoided as they can interfere with the absorption of the drugs. The overall NCCN statistics for this combination are:

Response Rate:

▶ PSA response in 40% to 60% of men.
▶ Soft tissue response in 45% to 55% of men.

Side Effects:

▶ Nausea.
▶ Hair loss (alopecia).
▶ Leukopenia (decrease in white blood cells) 25% of men.
▶ Blockage of the veins (deep vein thrombosis) in approximately 10% of men.

▶ Mitoxantrone (Novantrone®) and Prednisone®

This combination of drugs has focused on decreasing pain for men with hormone-refractory prostate cancer. In many studies using this combination, a high percentage of men experienced a complete response or partial response, meaning they had:

▶ A 50% decrease in pain medication (analgesic) use with no increase in pain.
▶ A decrease of 2 points on a 6-point pain scale, with no increase in analgesic use.

Serious side effects were limited to leukopenia (a decrease in the number of white blood cells that fight infection).

Because of these studies, the combination of Mitoxantrone/Prednisone® as a treatment for hormone-refractory prostate cancer has been approved by the Food and Drug Administration as a way to control pain in men with hormone-refractory prostate cancer. The overall NCCN statistics for this combination are:

Response Rate:

▶ PSA response in 33% of men.

▶ Palliative response (relief/comfort) in approximately 30% to 50% of men.

Side Effects:

▶ A small amount of nausea.

▶ Leukopenia (decrease in white blood cells) in 5% to 10% of men.

▶ Paclitaxel (Taxol®) and Estramustine

Paclitaxel and Estramustine have been shown to inhibit the way cancer cells divide. In one study looking at this combination, a PSA decrease of more than 50% was achieved in 53% of men. The combination is now being tested using a variety of dosage schedules, and early results seem promising. The overall NCCN statistics for this combination are:

Response Rate:

▶ PSA response in 53% of men.

▶ Soft tissue response in 44% of men.

Side Effects:

▶ Nausea.

▶ Breast enlargement (gynecomastia).

▶ Fluid retention.

▶ Leukopenia (decrease in white blood cells) in 20% of men.

▶ Estramustine and Docetaxel (Taxotere®)

The combination of Estramustine and Docetaxel has been demonstrated to be very effective at killing prostate cancer cells in preclinical models. In a recent study using this combination, 63% of the men had a drop in their PSA of greater than 50%, and a number of men were able to discontinue their use of pain medication. The results of multiple Phase II studies are available. (A Phase II study tests a specific regimen of drugs in a specific disease to find out the response rate.) Overall, the statistics for this combination are:

Response Rate:

▶ PSA response in 80% to 90% of men.

▶ Soft tissue response in 75% of men.

Side Effects:

▶ Edema (swelling in the legs).

▶ Fatigue.

▶ Esophagitis (inflammation of the esophagus that can be painful and make it temporarily difficult to eat).

▶ Cyclophosphamide (Cytoxan®), Diethylstilbestrol (DES), and Prednisone®

In a test of Cyclophosphamide (Cytoxan®), Diethylstilbestrol (DES), and Prednisone®, doctors looked at a group of men that had previously failed combined hormone therapy and had evidence of a rising PSA following antiandrogen withdrawal. Using this combination, almost 40% of these men showed a decrease in PSA of more than 50%. This combination was also well tolerated by men. Overall, the statistics for this combination are:

Response Rate:

▶ PSA response in 40% of men.

▶ Soft tissue response in 33% of men.

Side Effects:

▶ Minimal.

▶ Doxorubicin and Ketoconazole, Alternating with Vinblastine and Estramustine

The regimen of Doxorubicin and Ketoconazole, Alternating with Vinblastine and Estramustine has been tested extensively at the M.D. Anderson Cancer Center in Houston. The regimen is a bit difficult to follow because the treatment covers 56 days (more than twice as long as most other treatments), with each of the various drugs being given on certain days in the cycle. Side effects have been manageable. Overall, the statistics for this combination are:

Response Rate:

▶ PSA response in 67% of men.
▶ Soft tissue Response in 75% of men.

Side Effects:

▶ Edema or swelling in 50% of men.
▶ Deep vein thrombosis in 18% of men. (A deep venous thrombosis is a blood clot in the veins of the leg. This leads to swelling of the leg and the man then needs to be treated with a blood thinner such as Warfarin (trade name Coumadin®), generally for 6 months.)
▶ Cardiac problems in 4% of men.

THERAPIES ON THE HORIZON

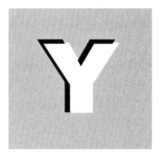

▶ Vaccines

One of the things that make treating cancer difficult is that the disease can hide from the immune system. The immune system consists of white blood cells (WBC) that recognize foreign substances or cells and destroy them. WBCs are also called leukocytes. They use the lymph nodes as their home bases to go out and fight infection. One type of WBC is called the neutrophil and it fights bacterial infections. Another kind of white blood cell, the lymphocyte, fights infection caused by viruses and destroys other cells, such as cancer cells, that are bad for the body.

This is accomplished in one of two ways:

▶ A subset of lymphocytes, the T cells, helps destroy cancer cells directly.

▶ A second subset of lymphocytes, the B cell, produces antibodies when it comes across a foreign cell. These antibodies attach to the cancer cell and tell another set of WBCs, the macrophages, that a bad cell is present, and they come to help destroy it.

Since T and B cells do not seem to recognize cancer cells very well, several researchers are trying to find and develop prostate cancer-specific antigens, or proteins, that will mark the cancer cells more effectively. They then inject these antigens under the skin and hope the immune system will recognize them as foreign and mount an immune response to them. This type of therapy is called a vaccine. Multiple vaccine trials are underway in the United States. In general, they are targeted at men with a rising PSA after failing local therapy such as a prostatectomy or prostatectomy + radiation. Some vaccine trials are open for men with hormone-refractory disease. Results from vaccine trials so far have been mixed. On the negative side, they only seem to help a small percentage of men. On the positive side, they have virtually no side effects. Vaccine trials, in general, open and close very quickly and it is difficult to predict which ones will be available at a given time. The good news is that doctors are developing better strategies to test all of the time.

▶ Gene Therapy

Another approach is gene therapy, which is currently available in several forms. In this approach, a gene is inserted into some of the lymphocytes, which changes them into far more effective cancer fighters. An alternate procedure inserts a gene that makes the cells "super attractors" for other cancer-fighting cells. These types of trials are still rare and it is more likely that various vaccine strategies will be used to unmask the immune system to fight cancer cells over the next several years.

There are currently three ways in which gene therapy may help men with prostate cancer:

- ▶ Establish a normal control of cell division, which could be done by inserting genes that suppress tumor development.
- ▶ Administer toxic products that target prostate cancer cells.
- ▶ Boost the immune system. This could be done by inserting tumor genes that the body recognizes as foreign, causing the immune system to kill all cancer cells related to the gene.

▶ Antibodies

Another way to use the immune system is to use antibodies. Cancer cells do express specific antigens or proteins on their cell surface that mark them as foreign to the body or specific to the cell type [like prostate-specific membrane antigen (PSMA)]. Several researchers are trying to isolate these antigens. When an antigen is isolated, an antibody to it will be made, which is another protein that binds to the antigen. The next part of the strategy is to attach a "radioactive bomb" to the antibody (such as radioactive iodine) and inject the combination into someone with the targeted cancer. These antibodies will then "home into" the cancer cells and destroy them with radioactivity. Antibody trials are still fairly rare, but should become more available over the next few years.

▶ Antiangiogenesis Therapy

New tumors often need blood to grow, so researchers hope that by reducing the growth of blood vessels feeding a tumor, they can reduce or stop its growth. Many angiogenesis inhibitors are being tested in clinical trials around the world. None have yet been approved for use in prostate cancer and all are considered experimental.

Angiostatin and Endostatin

Angiostatin and Endostatin are drugs that inhibit the growth of new blood vessels. Although early results in clinical trials have not been promising, they are being tested in multiple hospitals.

Thalidomide

Thalidomide has been known to be a potent inhibitor of blood vessel growth for many years. It was not used for many years because it was found to cause birth defects, however, it has been demonstrated to have some activity in treating men with hormone-refractory prostate cancer. Several clinical trials are ongoing with this drug, alone and in combination with other chemotherapy drugs. The major side effects of thalidomide appear to be fatigue and tingling of the fingers and toes (neuropathy).

▶ Anti-vascular Endothelial Growth Factor Inhibitors

Vascular endothelial growth factor (VEGF) is secreted by cancer cells to stimulate blood vessels to grow. Endothelial cells are the individual cells that line blood vessels. When VEGF binds to its receptor on endothelial cells it stimulates them to grow towards the tumor and feed it. Several inhibitors of the VEGF receptor are being tested. Many of these inhibitors are antibodies to the VEGF receptor itself.

▶ The Future

This is an exciting time in the development of new therapies for the treatment of advanced prostate cancer, and there are many clinical trials of advanced prostate cancers being conducted. These include trials sponsored by the National Cancer Institute (NCI) and drug companies. A good place to find information about clinical trials is at the various cancer center websites. Another source on the Internet is the NCI's trials list. The website is: http://www.nci.nih.gov/clinical_trials/. There are many websites on the Internet dedicated to prostate cancer—some of which advertise clinical trials. Support groups can also be a good source of information about such trials. See the Appendices for support groups and other helpful organizations.

▶ What about an Experimental Approach?

Someone considering any experimental procedure—or traditional treatment, for that matter—should ask the doctor six general questions:

- ▶ Can you describe the treatment?
- ▶ Who are the best candidates for this approach?
- ▶ How effective is this treatment and what are its side effects?
- ▶ How much does the treatment cost, and would my insurance cover it?
- ▶ What are its advantages?
- ▶ What are its disadvantages?

All treatments, drugs, and diagnostic tests are considered experimental unless they are approved by the U.S. Food and Drug Administration (FDA). The FDA appoints temporary advisory committees to advise an FDA drug review group. Members of these advi-

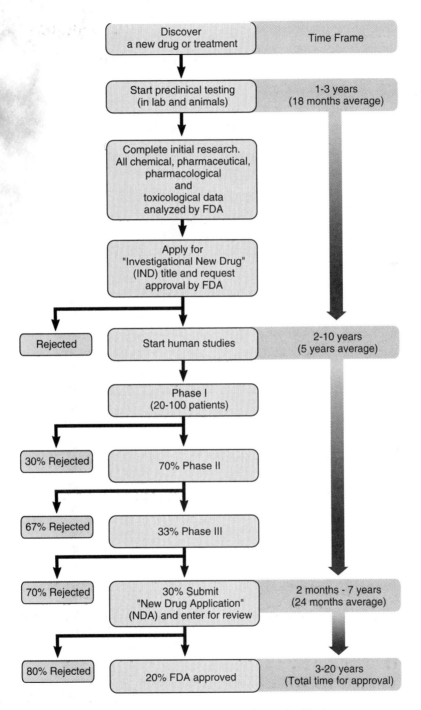

Source: *FDA Consumer Magazine, January 1995 (second edition)*

sory committees come from medical institutions, professional schools, government agencies, industry and trade associations, and consumer and patient groups nationwide.

The FDA approval process takes a long time, in some cases up to 20 years, because federal regulators require that a drug undergo rigorous testing and evaluation to ensure that it is safe and effective. In the late 1980s, however, the FDA introduced a faster approval system, but only for drugs or treatments that are used to treat life-threatening diseases. For example, under the older system, it took 21 years to approve Taxol®, a drug for ovarian cancer. Under the faster system, it took only 5 years to approve an AIDS drug called DDC.

When a procedure is not approved by the FDA it could mean one of the following:

▶ Not enough information or research is yet known about the procedure to determine whether it is effective and safe.

▶ The procedure is safe and effective but has yet to be approved by the FDA because it takes time to get approval.

▶ The procedure is not safe and effective but has yet to be disapproved by the FDA because this, too, takes time.

TREATMENT
OF
CANCER PAIN

Z

WHAT ARE SOME OF THE TREATMENTS FOR CANCER PAIN?

AN IMPORTANT PART OF DEALING WITH ADVANCED PROSTATE CANCER TREATMENT IS PALLIATIVE CARE, WHICH IS ESSENTIALLY ANY THERAPY THAT COMFORTS SOMEONE AND RELIEVES SYMPTOMS OF THE DISEASE. HORMONE ABLATION AND CHEMOTHERAPY ARE CONSIDERED EFFECTIVE FORMS OF PALLIATIVE THERAPY IN ADVANCED PROSTATE CANCER, BUT THERE ARE SEVERAL OTHER TREATMENTS AND DRUGS THAT MAY BE CALLED ON.

▶ Radiotherapy for Bone Pain

The majority of men with hormone-refractory disease have problems because their cancer has typically spread to the bones, where it can cause pain due to bone damage, bone fractures, and pressure on the bones from the expansion of the cancer. Pain can occur for a short time or it can be continuous, and the site of pain may move and change depending on activity or even changes in the weather.

▶ External-beam Radiation Therapy

External-beam radiation therapy in the form of local or "spot" radiation can be effective in controlling symptoms in a specific area. For example, if there is pain in one spot on the spine, then radiation can be given to that specific area to kill the cancer and relieve the pain. This is usually given in the form of 10 treatments of radiation in the space of approximately 2 weeks.

Nearly 80% of men with bone pain will experience at least partial pain relief with radiation treatment, and about 40% of men will have total pain relief. Side effects are relatively minor, and often depend on the site being treated. For example, radiation to the upper abdomen can cause nausea and vomiting, while radiation to the upper spine can lead to a sore throat or difficulty in swallowing. Such temporary symptoms can usually be treated with medication.

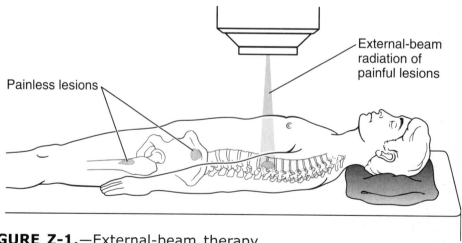

FIGURE Z-1.—External-beam therapy.

▶ Strontium-89 (Metastron®)

Another approach that has been the subject of much research is the use of injectable radiation or radioisotopes. One of these, Strontium-89, has been particularly well studied. Strontium-89 is effective because it follows the same path as calcium into the bones, but rather than settle into normal healthy bone, it goes to areas where the bone is changing, which tends to be the cancerous area. Cancerous bone actually absorbs strontium better than other tissues, so this may be why the majority of men feel better after just one injection. The effect is long-lasting, so the isotope can prevent pain caused by any additional cancer growth after the first injection. Strontium injections are given on the average of once every six months. They should not be given in intervals of less than 90 days.

Studies of Strontium-89 therapy show that:

▶ About 80% of men have pain relief with this type of therapy—typically, in 1 to 2 weeks.

▶ In the 80% of men who respond to Strontium-89, the effect lasts about 3 to 8 months—at which time another dose can be given.

▶ About 50% of men can expect to decrease their use of painkillers with this treatment. Strontium-89 can be given safely to those who have been previously treated with radiotherapy for relief of symptoms.

▶ Men treated with Strontium-89 in combination with radiotherapy had a significantly lower rate of developing new painful bone lesions, and those who developed new lesions had fewer of them.

▶ If the first injection is not helpful, then chances are that others will not be either.

The advantages of Strontium-89 therapy:

▶ It is as effective and more easily tolerated than spot radiation treatment for cancer pain.

▶ It is easy and fast to administer.

▶ It works only in the cancerous areas.

▶ The man is not a radiation hazard to others.

The disadvantages of Strontium-89 therapy:

▶ It can damage the bone marrow, which could cause a problem with blood clotting.

▶ It may cause short-term pain at the beginning of treatment, which is actually a good indicator of a better long-term result. The pain can be countered with other pain medications.

▶ Radioactive urine must be disposed in a special container for the first few days after injection.

If someone has kidney problems, the individual needs to be monitored carefully when receiving this treatment, because the Strontium-89 is radioactive, and excreted through the kidneys. For the same reason, men need to double-flush the toilet after urinating to make sure the slight amounts of radioactive material are taken away. The greatest potential side effect of Strontium-89 therapy, however, is a reduction in the number of platelets, which aid in clotting the blood. Thus, Strontium injections are given only after chemotherapy has been tried.

Samarium is a drug like Strontium-89 that is also being used. It does not damage the bone marrow cells as much as Strontium-89 and is gaining in popularity.

▶ Bisphosphonates

Some men with advanced prostate cancer may experience bone-pain relief from the use of diphosphonates (also called bisphosphonates). Bisphosphonates fight the breakdown of bone, and there are several clinical trials underway to see if these drugs are effective in blocking the spread of prostate cancer as well as in treating painful bone metastases. One recent study demonstrated that one such drug, zoledronic acid (Zometa®) decreased the amount of pain men were experiencing while on treatment for hormone refractory prostate cancer. In the study, half of the men were treated with chemotherapy alone, and the other half were treated with chemotherapy plus Zometa®. The men treated with the combination of chemotherapy and Zometa® used less narcotic pain medicine as well as experienced less breakage of bones (see figure). Zometa® has now been approved by the FDA for the treatment of bone metastases in men with advanced prostate cancer.

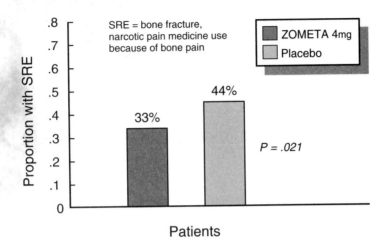

FIGURE Z-2.—Proportion of patients with Skeletal Related Event (SRE)

▶ Generalized Pain

There are too many medications that treat general body pain to discuss here. Someone experiencing generalized pain should talk to their doctor about the pain.

Over-the-Counter Medications and Prescription Drugs

If the pain is as bothersome as, say, a mild headache, the doctor may suggest an over-the-counter medication such as acetaminophen (Tylenol®) or ibuprofen (Motrin®), or one of the many prescription drugs for light pain. If the pain is constant and moderate or strong, then there are a number of possible narcotics that are effective, such as codeine and morphine. The key is to rate the pain (on a scale of 1 to 10, for example) so the doctor will know specifically how much pain someone is experiencing.

Do not be worry about narcotic addiction. There is no evidence to show that pain medications are addictive; in fact research has shown that pain management can increase the quality as well as the quantity of life.

Drug Patches. There are new ways pain medication can be delivered. One unique way is through a patch that is placed on the body. The patch can help those with strong or severe pain by releasing pain medication through the skin on a regular basis.

Wide-field Radiation. Also called "hemibody" radiation, this technique for managing generalized pain involves the use of radiation throughout the body.

The advantages of wide-field radiation:

▶ About half of men who undergo hemibody radiation experience partial or complete pain relief within 48 hours of treatment.

▶ Up to 80% of men feel relief within a week.

The disadvantages of wide-field radiation:

▶ It causes nausea and vomiting in 80% of those treated.

▶ It causes blood disorders in about 10% of men.

▶ Between 10% and 35% of men will experience inflammation of the lungs, a condition called radiation pneumonitis.

▶ Aspirin and Acetaminophen (Tylenol®)

Aspirin and Tylenol® are probably the most common over-the-counter pain medicines used. However, they are not very effective in treating bone pain related to prostate cancer.

▶ Nonsteroidal Anti-Inflammatory Drugs (NSAIDs)

Nonsteroidal Anti-Inflammatory Drugs (NSAIDs) are considered to be the first-line therapy for bone pain associated with prostate cancer. In reaction to the presence of cancer, the immune system tries to fight it by sending various white blood cells to the area where cancer is present. These white blood cells gather to fight the cancer cells directly (by attaching to them and killing them) as well as indirectly (by releasing chemicals called cytokines that attract other cells). This gathering of cells around the cancer is called inflammation. NSAIDs can help in treating bone pain because they stop the inflammation associated with cancer. They are primarily used for milder pain, and men who experience bone pain for the first time can be effectively treated with NSAIDs such as Ibuprofen. People react differently to medications, and may need to try more than one to find which one works best. The doctor may also recommend an "H2-blocker," which is a form of antacids that will help prevent any stomach upset from the NSAIDs.

Some of the Commonly Used NSAIDs

Voltaren Diflunisal®	Relafen®
Dolobid®	Naprosyn®
Advil®, Motrin®, Nuprin®	Alleve®
Indocin®	Feldene®
Toradol®	Clinoril®
Orudis®	Tolectin®

► Cyclo-oxygenase-2 (COX-2) Inhibitors

The cyclo-oxygenase-2 (COX-2) inhibitors are a new class of medicines that also act as an anti-inflammatory. The most common are Vioxx® and Celebrex®. These are often easier on the stomach than the traditional NSAIDs, but sometimes they can damage the kidneys so when you are taking these drugs it is not uncommon for the doctor to check how well your kidneys are working with a simple blood test.

► Narcotics

Narcotics are strong anti-pain medicines that work by blocking pathways in the brain that mediate pain called opiate receptors. They are used in addition to the NSAIDs. Many narcotics can be given either orally or via injection; one, known as Fentanyl®, can also be delivered through a patch. There are many different doses and forms of narcotics. They are available in weak and strong forms as well as short- and long-acting doses.

Commonly Used Narcotics

Morphine®	Percodan®
Codeine®	Dilaudid®
Fentanyl®	Methadone®

▶ Steroids

Steroids are another form of anti-inflammatory. They are also an effective therapy to treat bone pain. They work in a manner similar to NSAIDs; however, they can be associated with more side effects such as water retention and suppression of the immune system. At low dose, however, they are very safe. Different doctors use steroids at different times for the treatment of bone pain.

Commonly Used Steroids

Cortisone   Methylpredisolone®

Dexamethasone   Prednison®

Hydrocortisone

With all of the medicines and treatments available today, no man with prostate cancer should be in pain. There are simply too many good ways to get rid of it When used properly, narcotics do not lead to getting addicted. Men suffering from pain usually are because either they are too stubborn to take some pain medication as they are worried they will become addicted, or they are worried that it will make them dopey. Under appropriate supervision, these medicines and treatments are a wonderful boon to men with prostate cancer. No one should be afraid to ask for them.

Appendix
and
Glossary

APPENDIX

SUPPORT GROUPS AND OTHER HELPFUL ORGANIZATIONS

There is a lot of help available for men with prostate cancer and their loved ones. Below is an alphabetical summary of major national organizations that can put you in touch with support groups and other resources in your area.

American Cancer Society (ACS)
1599 Clifton Road, N.E.
Atlanta, GA 30329-4251
(800) ACS-2345
http://www.cancer.org

American Foundation for Urologic Disease (AFUD)
1128 North Charles Street
Baltimore, MD 21201
(410) 468-1800
(410) 468-1808 (fax)

American Institute for Cancer Research (AICR)
1759 R Street, N.W.
Washington, DC 20009
(800) 843-8114 (nutrition hotline)
(202) 328-7744
(202) 328-7226 (fax)
http://www.aicr.org
AICR is the only national cancer charity that focuses on the link between diet, nutrition, and cancer. AICR also provides information on breast, lung, colon, and prostate cancers.

American Urological Association (AUA)
1120 North Charles Street
Baltimore, MD 21201-5559
(410) 727-1100

Canadian Cancer Society
10 Alcorn Avenue, Suite 200
Toronto, Ontario, Canada M4V 3B1
Cancer Information Service toll-free
(888) 939-3333
(416) 961-7223
(416) 961-4189 (fax)

Cancer Care, Inc.
275 7th Avenue
New York, NY 10001
(800) 813-HOPE
(212) 302-2400
(212) 719-0263 (fax)
http://www.cancercare.org
Provides free professional counseling, support groups, and educational materials.

Cancer Research Institute
681 Fifth Avenue
New York, NY 10022
(800) 99-CANCER
(212) 688-7515
(212) 832-9376 (fax)
Supports leading cancer research.

CaPCURE, Inc.
1250 Fourth Street, Suite 360
Santa Monica, CA 90401
(800) 757-CURE
(310) 458-2873
(301) 458-8074 fax
capcure@capcure.org

CenterWatch: Clinical Trials Listing Service
http://www.centerwatch.com

CHEMOcare
231 North Avenue, West
Westfield, NJ 07090-1428
(800) 55-CHEMO
(908) 233-1103
(908) 233-0228 (fax)
Provides one-to-one emotional support to patients and families from trained and certified volunteers who themselves are cancer survivors.

Choice in Dying
1035 30th Street, N.W.
Washington, DC 20007
(800) 989-WILL
(202) 338-9790
(202) 338-0242 (fax)
http://www.partnershipforcaring.org
Provides counseling regarding preparing and using living wills and medical powers of attorney for health care.

CNN-Health
http://cnn.com/HEALTH/index.html

Coping Magazine
Copingmag@aol.com

Corporate Angel Network (CAN)
Westchester County Airport
One Loop Road
White Plains, NY 10604
(914) 328-1313
(914) 328-3938 (fax)

**Education Center for Prostate Cancer
   Patients (ECPCP)**
380 North Broadway, Suite 304
Jericho, NY 11753
(516) 942-5000
(516) 942-5025 (fax)

Families Against Cancer (FACT)
P.O. Box 588
DeWitt, NY 13214
(315) 446-6385
(315) 446-5326 (fax)
*FACT is an advocacy group for cancer
patients and their loved ones.*

Food and Drug Administration (FDA)
http://www.fda.gov

Geddings Obson Sr. Foundation
P.O. Box 1593
Augusta, GA 30903-1593
(800) 433-4215
http://www.impotence.org/
*Impotence education, services, and
support.*

Impotence Resource Center
P.O. Box 1593
Augusta, GA 30903

Incontinence on the Internet
http://incontinet.com

International Cancer Alliance (ICA)
4853 Cordell Avenue, Suite 11
Bethesda, MD 20814
(800) I-CARE-61
(301) 654-8684 (fax)
http://www.icare.org
*Provides a free Cancer Therapy Review,
which includes information on specific
types of cancer, from diagnosis to
treatment.*

Make Today Count
c/o Connie Zimmerman
Mid-America Cancer Center
1235 E. Cherokee
Springfield, MO 65804-2263
(800) 432-2273
(417) 888-7426 (fax)
*A mutual support organization for
cancer survivors.*

**Matthews Foundation for Prostate
   Cancer Research**
1142 Northeast 58th Street
Kirkland, WA 98033
(800) 234-6284
(425) 893-9657 (fax)
*Provides individual answers to prostate-
cancer survivors and their families about
the disease, its symptoms, and treatment.*

National Association for Continence (NAFC)

(used to be called Help for Incontinent People)
P.O. Box 8310
Spartanburg, SC 29305-8310
(800) BLADDER

National Association of Hospital Hospitality Houses Inc.

4013 W. Jackson Street
Muncie, IN 47304
(800) 542-9730
(317) 287-0321 (fax)
Provides information on lodging and support for those receiving medical care away from home.

National Cancer Institute

9000 Rockville Pike
Bethesda, MD 20892
(800) 532-4440
http://www.icic.nci.nih.gov
http://www.cancernet@icicc.nci.nih.gov

(800) 4-CANCER
Cancer Information Service:
A nationwide telephone service for cancer patients and their families, as well as the general public and health care professionals, that answers questions and provides free booklets about cancer.

(301) 402-5874
CancerFax:
Provides treatment summaries, with current data on prognosis, relevant staging and histologic classifications, news and announcements of important cancer-related issues.

National Cancer Survivors Day (NCSD) Foundation

P.O. Box 682285
Franklin, TN 37068-2285
(615) 794-3006
(615) 794-0179 (fax)
NCSD is a nationwide, annual celebration of life for cancer survivors, their loved ones, and health care professionals. NCSD is celebrated on the first Sunday in June throughout the United States.

National Coalition for Cancer Survivorship (NCCS)

1010 Wayne Avenue, Suite 505
Silver Spring, MD 20910
(301) 650-8868
(301) 565-9670 (fax)
Raises awareness of cancer survivorship through newsletters and other publications; provides education and advocacy for insurance, employment, and legal rights for those with cancer.

National Hospice Organization (NHO)

1700 Diagonal Road - Suite 300
Alexandria, VA 22314
(800) 658-8898
http:// www.nhpco.org

**National Institute on Aging
 Information Center**
P.O. Box 8057
Garthersburg, MD 20898-8057
(800) 222-2225

**National Kidney and Urologic
 Disease Information Clearinghouse**
Box NKUDIC
9000 Rockville Pike
Bethesda, MD 20892
(301) 654-4415
*For information on BPH and its
treatment.*

**National Prostate Cancer Coalition
 (NPCC)**
1156 15th Street, N.W., Suite 905
Washington, DC 20005
(202) 463-9455
(202) 463-9456 (fax)

The Oley Foundation
214 Hun Memorial
Albany Medical Center A-23
Albany, NY 12208
(800) 776-OLEY
(518) 262-5079
(518) 262-5528 (fax)
*Support for those who require home
parenteral and/or enteral nutrition.*

OncoLink
http://cancer.med.upenn.edu

**Patient Advocates for Advanced
 Cancer Treatments (PAACT)**
1143 Parmalee, N.W.
Grand Rapids, MI 49504
(616) 453-1477
(616) 453-1846 (fax)

**Prostate Cancer Research &
 Education Foundation (PC-REF)**
6699 Alvarado Road, Suite 2301
San Diego, CA 92120
(619) 287-8866

**Prostate Cancer Resource Institute
 (PCRI)**
5777 West Century Blvd., Suite 885
Los Angeles, CA 90045
(310) 743-2110
(310) 743-2113 (fax)

**Prostate Cancer Support Group
 Network (PCSN)**
300 W. Pratt Street, Suite 401
Baltimore, MD 21201
(800) 828-7866

Prostate Health Council
c/o American Foundation for Urologic
 Disease Inc. (AFUD)
300 W. Pratt Street, Suite 401
Baltimore, MD 21201-2463
(800) 242-2383

R.A. Bloch Cancer Foundation, Inc.
The Cancer Hotline
4410 Main Street
Kansas City, MO 64111
(816) 932-8453
(816) 931-7486 (fax)
Provides information, peer counseling, medical second opinions, and support groups for those with cancer.

Robert Benjamin Ablin Foundation for Cancer Research
115 Franklin Turnpike, Suite 200
Mahwah, NJ 07430
(973) 248-9395
http://www.prostatefoundation.org
The Robert Benjamin Ablin Foundation for Cancer Research is directed toward development and improvement of methods of early detection, diagnosis, and treatment of prostate cancer.

Ronald McDonald House
Ronald McDonald House Charities
1 Kroc Drive
Oak Brook, IL 60521
(630) 623-7048
(630) 623-7488 (fax)
Offers lodging for family members of cancer patients being treated away from home.

Sex Information and Education Council of the U.S.
130 W. 42nd Street
New York, NY 10036
(212) 819-9770

The Oley Foundation
http://www.oley.org
Support for those who require home parenteral and/or enteral nutrition.

The Simon Foundation for Continence
P.O. Box 815
Wilmette, IL 60091
(800) 23-SIMON

The Wellness Community
2716 Ocean Park Blvd., Suite 1040
Santa Monica, CA 90405-5211
(310) 314-2555
(310) 314-7586 (fax)
Provides free psychosocial support to cancer survivors through 16 facilities nationwide.

U.S. Department of Health and Human Services
Public Health Service Agency for Health Care Policy and Research Publications Clearinghouse
P.O. Box 8547
Silver Springs, MD 20907
(800) 358-9295
To get a copy of BPH health guidelines.

U.S. Food and Drug Administration (FDA)
Drug Information Branch—HFD210
5600 Fishers Lane
Rockville, MD 20857
(301) 827-4573

US TOO International, Inc.
930 North York Road, Suite 50
Hinsdale, IL 60521-2993
(800) 808-7866
(630) 323-1002
(630) 323-1003 (fax)

NOTES

GLOSSARY

Abdomen

The abdomen is the part of the body below the ribs and above the pelvic bone that contains organs like the intestines, liver, kidneys, stomach, bladder, and prostate.

Abdominal-Pelvic CT
  (computed tomography) Scan

An abdominal-pelvic CT (computed tomography) scan is an X-ray scan that images the various organs in the abdomen and pelvis. It is used to determine whether the pelvic lymph nodes have been affected with prostate cancer.

Ablation

Ablation means reduction of; for example, in the management of prostate cancer, the killing off of cancer cells by radiation, cryotherapy, hormonal therapy, or chemotherapy.

Acid Phosphatase

Acid phosphatase, which is also called *prostate-acid phosphatase* (PAP), is a substance produced and released by the prostate; higher levels can indicate prostate cancer. Before the *prostate-specific antigen* (PSA) test was developed, a test that measured acid-phosphatase levels was used to detect prostate cancer. While the PSA test is a superior method of cancer detection, some doctors still use the acid-phosphatase test along with PSA to help determine whether cancer has spread beyond the prostate. The normal level for acid phosphatase varies according to the type of assay, or test, used.

Acute Bacterial Prostatitis

Acute bacterial prostatitis is a form of prostatitis (inflammation of the prostate) that is caused by bacteria. Symptoms include painful and difficult urination, pain in the lower back and perineum (area between the scrotum and anus), chills, fever, and blood in the urine. This type of prostatitis is usually associated with a urinary tract infection (UTI).

Adenocarinoma

Adenocarinoma is a form of cancer that develops from a malignant abnormality in the cells lining a glandular organ such as the prostate; almost all prostate cancers are adenocarcinomas.

Adjuvant Therapy

Adjuvant therapy is an additional treatment used to increase the effectiveness of the primary therapy; radiation therapy and hormonal therapy are often used as adjuvant treatments following a radical prostatectomy.

Adrenal Androgens

The adrenal glands, which sit on top of the kidneys, produce small amounts of male hormones (androgens), including testosterone. While about 95% of testosterone is produced by the testicles, about 5% to 10% comes from the adrenal glands. The effect of adrenal hormones on prostate cancer is unknown. Some physicians think they can contribute to the spread of prostate cancer while others think that the quantity is not large enough to be of concern. (On the other hand, there is no question that testosterone from the testicles can increase the growth

rate of prostate cancer; this is why many men are treated with antiandrogens and why many men with advanced prostate disease have their testicles removed.)

Adrenal Glands

The two adrenal glands are located above the kidneys. They produce a variety of different hormones, including sex hormones, the adrenal androgens make about 5% to 10% of circulating testosterone.

Adrenalectomy

Adrenalectomy is the surgical removal of one or both adrenal glands.

Adriamycin

Adriamycin is a chemotherapy agent for advanced prostate cancer.

Age-Adjusted

A result that takes into account the age of an individual or group of individuals is age-adjusted. For example, prostate cancer survival data and average normal PSA values can be adjusted according to the ages of groups of men.

Age- and Race-Specific PSA Reference Ranges

PSA level tends to rise with age, and a man's racial background can also affect his normal PSA level. This concept has led to the widespread use of age- and race-specific reference ranges for determining normal PSA levels. So, although the traditional normal PSA range is between 0-4 ng/ml, the upper limit of normal can be as low as 2.5 ng/ml or as high as 6.5 ng/ml, depending on a man's age and race.

Alkaline Phosphatase
Alkaline phosphatase is an enzyme in blood, bone, kidney, spleen and lungs. An alkaline phosphatase test is used to detect bone or liver metastasis.

Alpha-Blockers
Alpha-blockers are drugs that act on the prostate by relaxing certain types of muscle tissue. These drugs are often used in the treatment of BPH, but not in the treatment of cancer.

Analgesic
An analgesic is a type of medicine or a form of treatment that relieves pain.

Analog (analogue)
Analog (analogue) is a synthetic chemical, or pharmaceutical, that behaves very like a normal chemical in the body, e.g. LHRH analogs.

Anandron
Anandron is the trade or brand name for nilutamide, an antiandrogen.

Anastomosis
An anastomosis is the place where two different structures are surgically reattached or reconnected after an organ has been re-moved. For example, during radical prostatectomy (removal of the prostate) the neck of the bladder and the urethra are recon-nected, or "anastomosed."

Androcur
Androcur is the trade name for cyproter-one, an antiandrogen.

Androgen
An androgen is a hormone that is respon-sible for male characteristics and the de-velopment and function of male sexual or-gans (e.g., testosterone) produced mainly by the testicles but also in the cortex of the adrenal glands.

Androgen Ablation
Another name for hormone therapy. The loss of testosterone as a result of surgical or medical castration.

Androgen-Dependent (hormone-sensitive) Cells
Androgen-dependent (hormone-sensitive) cells are prostate =cancer cells that depend on hormones to survive, or grow. When their hormonal supply is cut off these cells have trouble functioning. The higher a tumor's percentage of hormone-sensitive cells, the better it will respond to treatment with hormone-blocking therapy.

Androgen Deprivation
See androgen ablation

Androgen-Independent (hormone-insensitive) Cells

Androgen-independent (hormone-insensitive) cells are prostate-cancer cells that do not depend on hormones to survive, or grow. These are more difficult prostate-cancer cells to deal with because anti-androgen therapy does not work on them. The higher a tumor's percentage of hormone-insensitive cells, the less likely it will respond to treatment.

Androgen Receptors

Testosterone binds to androgen receptors inside the prostate cells. After binding, it causes growth of the cells.

Aneuploid

Aneuploid is a term that refers to fast-growing cancer cells. (Also see flow cytometry.)

Anesthetic

An anesthetic is a drug that produces general or local loss of physical sensations, particularly pain. For example, a "spinal" is the injection of a local anesthetic into the area surrounding the spinal cord.

Aneuploid

Aneuploid is having an abnormal number of sets of chromosomes. For example, tetraploid means having two paired sets of chromosomes, which is twice as many as normal.

Angiogenesis

Angiogenesis is the formation of new blood vessels; a characteristic of tumors.

Anterior

Anterior, or the front; for example, the anterior of the prostate faces forward.

Antiandrogen

An antiandrogen is a compound (usually a synthetic pharmaceutical) that blocks or otherwise interferes with the normal action of androgens at cellular receptor sites.

Antiandrogen Withdrawal Response (AAWR)

Antiandrogen withdrawal response (AAWR) is a decrease in PSA caused by the withdrawal of an antiandrogen such as flutamide (Eulexin), bicalutamide (Casodex), or nilutamide (Anadron) after combined hormonal therapy (CHT) begins to fail. It occurs when there are PCa cells that have mutated to feed on the anti-androgen rather than on testosterone (T) or dihydrotestosterone (DHT).

Antiandrogen Therapy

See Hormonal Therapy.

Antibiotic

An antibiotic is a drug that can kill certain types of bacteria.

Antibody
An antibody is a protein produced by the immune system as a defense against an invading or "foreign" material or substance (an antigen). For example, when someone gets a cold their body produces antibodies to the cold virus.

Anticholinergic Drugs
Anticholinergic drugs are medications that can be used to treat urinary incontinence.

Anticoagulant
An anticoagulant is a drug that helps to stop the blood from clotting. Heparin, Coumadin®, and aspirin are just three of many drugs that prevent blood from clotting. Such drugs should be avoided before surgery to prevent blood loss.

Antigen
An antigen is "foreign" material introduced into the body (a virus or bacterium, for example) or other material that the immune system considers to be foreign because it is not part of the body's normal biology (e.g., prostate cancer cells). An antibody is the immune system's response to an antigen.

Anus
The anus is the opening of the rectum.

Apex
The apex is the tip or bottom of the prostate gland, e.g., the part of the prostate farthest away from the bladder.

Artificial Sphincter
An artificial sphincter is an implantable device used to treat urinary incontinence (loss of urinary control) that has persisted for a year or more.

Aspirin
See Anticoagulant.

Aspiration
Aspiration is the use of suction to remove fluid or tissue, usually through a fine needle (e.g., aspiration biopsy).

Assay
An assay is a test that measures the amount of a certain substance in the body. For example, a PSA test is also called a PSA assay.

Asymptomatic
Asymptomatic is having no recognizable symptoms of a particular disorder.

Atypical Adenomatous Hyperplasia (AAH)
A change in the way the cells and glands of the prostate look. It is unclear if this is associated with cancer.

Autodonation of Blood

Autodonation (or autologous donation) of blood is when someone banks their own blood in case a transfusion is needed at a later date. Men who are planning to undergo radical prostatectomy (surgical removal of the prostate) are often advised to bank their blood in case they experience some blood loss during the operation.

Autologous

Autologous is one's own. For example, autologous blood is someone's own blood that is removed prior to surgery and banked in case a transfusion is needed during or after surgery.

B

Balloon Dilation

Balloon dilation is a treatment for benign prostatic hyperplasia (BPH) that is no longer frequently used. During balloon dilation, a tiny, deflated balloon is placed through a catheter into the portion of the urethra that runs through the prostate. The balloon is then inflated, which stretches the urethra and allows urine to flow more easily from the bladder. The balloon is then deflated and removed.

Base

The base of the prostate gland is the wide part at the top of the prostate closest to the bladder.

Benign

Benign is relatively harmless; not cancerous; not malignant.

Benign Prostate Hyperplasia (or hypertrophy) (BPH)

Benign prostate hyperplasia (or hypertrophy) (BPH) is a noncancerous condition of the prostate that results in the growth of both glandular and stromal (supporting connective) tissue, enlarging the prostate and obstructing urination.

Benign Prostatic Hypertrophy (BPH)

Benign prostatic hypertrophy (BPH) is similar to benign prostatic hyperplasia, but caused by an increase in the size of cells rather than the growth of more cells.

Bicalutamide

Bicalutamide (the trade name is Casodex®) is a nonsteroidal antiandrogen available in the United States and some European countries for the treatment of prostate cancer.

Bilateral

Bilateral is both sides. For example, a bilateral orchiectomy is a procedure in which both testicles are removed and a bilateral adrenalectomy is an operation in which both adrenal glands are removed.

Bilateral Orchiectomy

Bilateral orchiectomy is the surgical removal of the testicles, also called surgical castration. This procedure stops the body from producing large amounts of testosterone, which in turn slows the growth of prostate cancer. This procedure is only used in men whose cancer has spread beyond the prostate.

Biopsy

Biopsy is the sampling of tissue from a particular part of the body (e.g., the prostate) in order to check for abnormalities such as cancer. In the case of prostate cancer, biopsies are usually carried out under ultrasound guidance using a specially designed device known as a prostate biopsy gun; removed tissue is typically examined microscopically by a pathologist in order to make a precise diagnosis.

Bisphosphonates

Medicines that are used to prevent bone density loss.

Bladder

The bladder is the hollow organ in which urine is collected and stored.

Bladder Neck

The bladder neck is the part of the bladder that opens into the urethra and allows urinary control. Input from the brain can either relax the bladder-neck muscles so that urine can flow out of the bladder and into the urethra (so someone can urinate), or tighten the bladder neck so that urine can remain in the bladder.

Bladder-Neck Contracture

A bladder-neck contracture is a complication of surgery in which the bladder neck is scarred. This can cause future urinary problems that may require surgical repair.

Blood Chemistry

Blood chemistry measures concentrations of many chemicals in the blood; abnormal values can indicate spread of cancer or side effects of therapy.

Blood Count

A blood count is the analysis of blood cells and platelets; abnormal values can indicate cancer in the bone or the side effects of therapy.

Blood-Thinning Drugs

See Anticoagulant.

Bone Marrow

Bone marrow is soft tissue in bone cavities that produces blood cells.

Bone Scan

A bone scan is a technique more sensitive than conventional X-rays that uses a radio-labeled agent to identify abnormal or cancerous growths within or attached to bone. In the case of prostate cancer, a bone scan is used to identify bony metastases that are definitive for cancer that has escaped from the prostate. Metastases appear as "hot spots" on the film. However, the absence of hot spots does not prove the absence of tiny metastases. Bone scans can also be positive because of old injuries or arthritis.

Bowel Preparation
Bowel preparation is the cleaning of the bowels or intestines, which is normal prior to abdominal surgery such as radical prostatectomy.

BPH
See Benign Prostate Hyperplasia.

Brachytherapy
Brachytherapy is a form of radiation therapy in which radioactive seeds or pellets that emit radiation are implanted in order to kill surrounding tissue (e.g., the prostate, including prostate cancer cells).

C

Cancer
Cancer is the growth of abnormal cells in the body in an uncontrolled manner. Unlike benign tumors, these tend to invade surrounding tissues and spread to distant sites of the body via the bloodstream and lymphatic system.

Capsule
The fibrous tissue that acts as an outer lining of the prostate is known as the capsule.

Carcinoma
Carcinoma is a form of cancer that originates in tissues that line or cover a particular organ (see Adenocarcinoma).

Carcinosarcoma
Carcinosarcoma is a rare tumor of the prostate that is made up of epithelial (carcino) and connective tissue (sarcoma) components. It usually has a poor prognosis.

Cardura®
See Alpha-Blockers.

Casodex®
Casodex® is a brand or trade name of bicalutamide.

Castration
Castration is the use of surgical or medical techniques to eliminate testosterone produced by the testes.

Catheter
A catheter is a hollow (usually flexible plastic) tube that can be used to drain fluids from or inject fluids into the body. In the case of prostate cancer, it is common for men to have a transurethral catheter to drain urine for some time after treatment by surgery or some forms of radiation therapy.

CAT Scan
See Computerized Axial Tomography.

CDUS
See Color-Flow Doppler Ultrasound.

Central Zone (CZ)
The central zone is one of the four zones of the prostate. Only 5% to 10% of prostate cancers begin in this area. The other three zones are called the periurethral zone, the transition zone, and the peripheral zone.

Chemotherapy
Chemotherapy is the use of drugs or other chemicals to kill cancer cells.

Chemotherapeutic Drugs
Chemotherapeutic drugs are a variety of drugs that can kill cancer cells.

Chromagranin A (CGA)
Chromagranin A (CGA) is a small cell prostate cancer or neuroendocrine cell marker.

Chronic Bacterial Prostatitis
Chronic bacterial prostatitis is a type of prostatitis, or inflammation of the prostate, caused by bacteria. It is associated with chronic urinary tract infections (UTIs). Symptoms include painful, difficult, and frequent urination; and pain in the lower back, penis, perineum (area between the scrotum and anus) and/or pubic area.

Clinical Staging of Prostate Cancer
Clinical staging is an estimation of the stage, or severity, of prostate cancer based on the results of the PSA blood test, the digital rectal exam, the transrectal ultrasound, and prostate biopsy.

Clinical Trial
A clinical trial is a carefully planned experiment to evaluate a treatment or a medication (often a new drug) for an unproven use. Phase I trials are very preliminary short-term trials involving a few people to see if drugs have any activity or any serious side effects. Phase II trials may involve 20 to 50 people and are designed to estimate the most active dose of a new drug and determine its side effects. Phase III trials involve many people and compare a new therapy against the current standard or best available therapy.

Color-Flow Doppler Ultrasound (CDUS)
Color-flow Doppler ultrasound (CDUS) is an ultrasound method that more clearly images tumors by observing the Doppler shift in sound waves caused by the rapid flow of blood through tiny blood vessels that are characteristic of tumors.

Combination Hormone Blockade (CHB)
Combination hormone blockade (CHB) is the same as combined hormonal therapy (CHT) or androgen deprivation therapy (ADT) or maximal androgen blockade (MAB). It usually involve an LHRH agonist and an antiandrogen.

Combined, or Double-Agent, Androgen-Deprivation Therapy

Combined, or double-agent, androgen-deprivation therapy is the use of an antiandrogen with an orchiectomy or an LHRH agonist to interfere with the cancer cells ability to interact with testosterone. Also called complete hormonal therapy (CHT), this treatment appears to have an advantage over single-agent androgen deprivation therapy, especially when used for prostate cancer that has just spread locally beyond the prostate (stage C or T3).

Combined Hormonal Therapy (CHT)

Combined hormonal therapy (CHT) is the use of more than one hormone in therapy; especially the use of LHRH analogs (e.g., Lupron®, Zoladex®) to block the production of testosterone by the teslus es, plus antiandrogens [e.g., Eulexin® (flutamide), Casodex® (bicalutamide), Anadron (nilutamide), Androcur® (Cyproterone)], to compete with DHT and T (testosterone) for cell sites, thereby depriving cancer cells of DHT and T needed for growth.

Complication

A complication is an unexpected or unwanted effect of a treatment, drug, or other procedure.

Complete Androgen Blockade (CAB)

See Combined Hormonal Therapy.

Complete Hormonal Therapy (CHT)

See Combined, or Double-Agent, Androgen-Deprivation Therapy.

Computed Tomography Scan

Computed tomography scan is also called a CT, or CAT, scan. This involves a large number of X-rays which, when stacked together, provide a three-dimensional, cross-sectional view of certain structures in the body. It helps some doctors with prostate-cancer staging. It also can assist in more accurate delivery of external-beam radiation by determining the exact position of the prostate.

Computerized Axial Tomography

Computerized axial tomography (also known as CT scan and CAT scan) is a method of combining images from multiple X-rays under the control of a computer to produce cross-sectional or three-dimensional pictures of the internal organs, which can be used to identify abnormalities. It can identify prostate enlargement, but is not always effective for assessing the stage of prostate cancer. However, for evaluating metastases of the lymph nodes or more distant soft tissue sites, the CAT scan is significantly more accurate.

Concurrent

At the same time. This usually refers to when two therapies, like radiation and hormones, are given at the same time.

Conformational Therapy

Conformational therapy is the use of careful planning and delivery techniques designed to focus radiation on the areas of the prostate and surrounding tissue that need treatment and to protect areas that do not need treatment. Three-dimensional conformational therapy is a more sophisticated form of this method.

Contracture

A contracture is scarring that can occur at the bladder neck after a radical prostatectomy and which results in narrowing of the passage between the bladder and the urethra.

Core

A core is a piece of tissue taken during a biopsy procedure. All prostate biopsies should involve taking at least six different cores, also called a sextant biopsy.

Corpora Cavernosa

The corpora cavernosa is the part of a man's penis that fills with blood when he is sexually excited.

Corpora Spongiosum

The corpora spongiosum is a spongy chamber in a man's penis that fills with blood when he is sexually excited.

Cryoablation

Cryoablation is also called cryotherapy or cryosurgery. It involves the use of very low temperatures to freeze the prostate and thus kill prostate-cancer cells and/or stop the cancer from growing. The low temperatures are achieved through the use of liquid nitrogen.

Cryosurgery

Cryosurgery is the use of liquid nitrogen probes to freeze a particular organ to extremely low temperatures to kill the tissue, including any cancerous tissue. When used to treat prostate cancer, the cryoprobes are guided by transrectal ultrasound.

Cryotherapy

See Cryosurgery.

CT Scan, Computerized or Computed Tomography

See Computerized Axial Tomography.

Cyclophosphamide (Cytoxan®)

Cyclophosphamide (Cytoxan®) is an oral chemotherapy agent that can be used in the treatment of advanced prostate cancer.

Cyproterone

Cyproterone is an antiandrogen.

Cyst

Cyst is the prefix for bladder. For example, cystoscopy means viewing the bladder with a device.

Cystitis

Cystitis is an inflammation of the bladder, which often causes painful urination. This can be a side effect of radiation therapy or simply the result of a bacterial infection of the bladder.

Cystometry

Cystometry is a procedure in which a tiny catheter is threaded through the urethra into a full bladder to measure the organ's function and pressure.

Cystoscope

Cystoscope is an instrument used by physicians to look inside the bladder and the urethra.

Cystoscopy

Cystoscopy is the use of a cystoscope to view the bladder, prostate, and urethra.

Cytokines

Cytokines are growth factors important to cellular function, they help normal and cancer cells grow.

CZ

See Central Zone (CZ).

D

Debulking

Debulking is the reduction of the volume of cancer by one of several techniques; most frequently used to imply surgical debulking.

DES

See Diethylstilbestrol.

Dexamethasone (Decadron)

Dexamethasone (Decadron) is a high-dose steroid usually given if it is suspected that someone may have a spinal cord compression.

DHT

See Dihydrotestosterone.

Diagnosis

A diagnosis is the evaluation of signs, symptoms, and selected test results by a physician to determine the physical and biological causes of the signs and symptoms and whether a specific disease or disorder is involved.

DIC

See Disseminated Intravascular Coagulation.

Diethylstilbestrol (DES)

Diethylstilbestrol (DES) is a female hormone commonly used in treatment of prostate cancer.

Differentiation

Differentiation is the use of the differences between prostate cancer cells when seen under the microscope as a method to grade the severity of the disease. Well differentiated cells are easily recognized as normal cells, while poorly differentiated cells are abnormal, cancerous, and difficult to recognize as belonging to any particular type of cell group.

Digital Rectal Examination (DRE)

Digital rectal examination (DRE) is the use by a physician of a lubricated and gloved finger inserted into the rectum to feel for abnormalities of the prostate and rectum.

Dihydrotestosterone

Dihydrotestosterone (DHT) (5-alpha-dihydrotestosterone) is the male hormone that is most active in the prostate. It is manufactured when an enzyme (5-alpha-reductase) in the prostate stimulates the transformation of testosterone to DHT.

Diploid

Diploid is having one complete set of normally paired chromosomes (i.e., a normal amount of DNA). Diploid cancer cells tend to grow slowly and respond well to hormone therapy.

Disseminated Intravascular Coagulation

Disseminated intravascular coagulation (DIC) is a blood-clotting disorder that can occur in some men with advanced prostate cancer.

Disseminated Prostate Cancer

Disseminated prostate cancer is cancer that is found throughout the prostate or throughout the body. This is the opposite of focal prostate cancer, which is found only in one area of the gland.

Diuretics

Diuretics are drugs that rid the body of excess water through more frequent urination.

DNA

Deoxyribonucleic acid (DNA) is the basic biologically active chemical that defines the physical development and growth of nearly all living organisms.

Docetaxel (Taxotere®)

Docetaxel (Taxotere®) is a chemotherapy agent for hormone-refractory prostate cancer. It is a microtubule inhibitor. It is often used with estramustine.

Double-Agent Androgen-Deprivation Therapy

See Combined, or Double-Agent, androgen-Deprivation Therapy.

Double-Blind Study

A double-blind study is a form of clinical trial in which neither the physician nor the individual know the actual treatment that anyone is receiving. Double-blind trials are a way of minimizing the effects of the personal opinions of individuals and physicians on the results of the trial.

Doubling Time

Doubling time is the time that it takes a particular focus of cancer to double in size.

Dorsal Vein Complex
The veins near the prostate.

Downsizing
Downsizing is the use of hormonal or other forms of management to reduce the volume of prostate cancer in and/or around the prostate prior to attempted curative treatment.

Downstaging
Downstaging is the use of hormonal or other forms of management in the attempt to lower the clinical stage of prostate cancer prior to attempted curative treatment (e.g., from stage T3a to stage T2b). This technique is highly controversial.

Doxazosin
See Alpha-Blockers.

DRE
See Digital Rectal Examination.

Dry Ejaculation
Dry ejaculation is a condition, also called retrograde ejaculation, in which semen does not come out of the penis when a man has an orgasm. Instead, the semen flows back into the bladder because the bladder neck is damaged. Dry ejaculation is a complication of transurethral resection and other various prostate procedures.

Ductal Carcinoma
Ductal carcinoma is a rare tumor of the prostate that begins growing in a prostate duct (ducts are locations of excretions or secretions from a gland, for example the periurethral duct/glands of the prostate). The prognosis of this cancer varies from good to poor.

Dysplasia
See PIN.

Dysuria
Dysuria is urination that is problematic or painful.

E

Edema
Edema is swelling or accumulation of fluid in some part of the body.

Ejaculation
Ejaculation is the discharging of semen from the penis during orgasm. Semen, also called ejaculate, is made up of sperm cells and fluid produced by a variety of reproductive organs, including the prostate.

Ejaculatory Ducts
Ejaculatory ducts are the tubular passages through which semen reaches the prostatic urethra during orgasm.

Emcyt®

Emcyt® is the brand or trade name of estramustine phosphate in the United States.

Endogenous

Endogenous is inherent, naturally to the organism.

Enucleate

Enucleate is usually used in conjunction with prostate-removal surgery, in which the surgeon's fingers are used to remove, or enucleate, prostatic tissue from around the urethra.

Epididymis

The epididymis is where sperm is stored after it is made in the testicles. It is where sperm cells begin to mature and acquire the ability to swim, or move.

Epidural Anesthesia

Epidural anesthesia is the injection of anesthetic into the spine through a thin tube. After the initial dose, additional anesthetic can be given as needed to numb the lower body. The amount of pain relief and the area of numbness can be adjusted with this form of anesthesia, during which the individual remains conscious.

Erectile Dysfunction

Erectile dysfunction is when an erection is not strong enough for sexual intercourse to occur.

Estramustine Phosphate

Estramustine phosphate is a chemotherapeutic agent used in the treatment of some men with advanced prostate cancer.

Estrogen

Estrogen is a female hormone; certain estrogens (e.g., diethylstilbestrol) are used by some physicians for treatment of prostate cancer. Also made in small quantities in males, especially as they age. Estrogens are used to block testosterone production in men with advanced prostate cancer. The most commonly used estrogen is diethylstilbestrol (DES), which is taken orally.

Etoposide

Etoposide (VP-16, VePesid®) is an oral chemotherapy drug that is used for the treatment of hormone-refractory prostate cancer. It is used in conjunction with estramustine.

Eulexin®

Eulexin® is an antiandrogen used in the treatment of prostate cancer. Made by Schering, it is also known by the generic name flutamide.

Experimental

An unproven (or even untested) technique or procedure is known as experimental. Certain experimental treatments are commonly used in the management of prostate cancer.

External Radiation Therapy (also External-Beam Therapy)

External radiation therapy (also external-beam therapy) is a treatment for prostate cancer in which a high dose of radiation is delivered from an outside source (hence the name external) into the prostate to kill the cancer and stop it from growing. This treatment requires someone to come to the hospital five days a week for four to six weeks. Each treatment session lasts about 15–30 minutes.

Extracapsular Prostate Tissue

Extracapsular prostate tissue is the tissue that immediately surrounds the outside, or capsule, of the prostate. Cancer that has spread to this area and beyond is considered to be advanced disease.

F

False Negative

A false negative is an erroneous negative test result. For example, an imaging test that fails to show the presence of a cancer tumor, later found by biopsy, is said to have returned a false negative result.

False Positive

A false positive is a positive test result mistakenly identifying a state or condition that does not in fact exist.

FDA

See Food and Drug Administration.

Finasteride

Finasteride an antiandrogen drug, made by Merck, is known by the trade name Proscar®. It is an inhibitor of the enzyme 5-alpha-reductase, which converts testosterone into dihydrotestosterone (DHT), a more powerful form of testosterone). Finasteride also shows promise in preventing prostate cancer and promoting hair growth; its effectiveness in these areas is currently being evaluated. Used to treat BPH.

Five-alpha-Reductase

Five-alpha-reductase (5-alpha-reductase) is an enzyme in the prostate that can convert testosterone into a stronger form of testosterone called dihydrotestosterone (DHT).

Five-alpha-Reductase Inhibitors

Five-alpha reductase (5-alpha-reductase) inhibitors are a type of drug that prevents the conversion of testosterone to dihydrotestosterone (DHT). Prosca®r (finasteride), made by Merck, is one of these inhibitors and it is used in the treatment of benign prostate enlargement and in the National Prostate Cancer Prevention Trial.

Flare Reaction

A flare reaction is a temporary increase in tumor growth and symptoms caused by

LHRH agonists. It can be mild to dangerous but may be prevented by taking an antiandrogen (generally Casodex® or Eulexin®) several days before starting a LHRH agonist (Lupron® or Zoladex®).

Flow Cytometry

Flow cytometry is a technique that identifies the genetic makeup of cancerous cells as diploid (slow-growing), aneuploid or polyploid (aggressive, or fast-growing).

Fluoroscopy

Fluoroscopy is a moving X-ray image that appears live on a screen as opposed to waiting to see an actual photograph or film. It is used most commonly for viewing the lower urinary tract before and after treatment.

Flutamide

Flutamide (Eulexin®) is an antiandrogen used in the palliative hormonal treatment of advanced prostate cancer and sometimes in the adjuvant and neoadjuvant hormonal treatment of earlier stages of prostate cancer; normal dosage is 2 capsules every 8 hours (not just at meals).

Focal Prostate Cancer

Focal prostate cancer is found in only one or a few small areas of the prostate.

Foley Catheter

A Foley catheter is a tube that is inserted into the urethra and bladder through the tip of the penis. In addition to draining urine from the bladder, it can be used to irrigate the bladder and prostatic urethra to prevent the formation of blood clots.

Follicle-Stimulating Hormone (FSH)

Follicle-stimulating hormone (FSH) is a hormone that stimulates sperm production in the testicles.

Following Expectantly

Following expectantly is an uncommon terminology for watchful waiting, the practice of monitoring the course of prostate cancer without immediately pursuing active treatment.

Food and Drug Administration (FDA)

The Food and Drug Administration (FDA) is a federal agency that approves drugs and treatments for public use. The approval criteria deal with issues of safety and treatment effectiveness.

Frequency

Frequency is the need to urinate often.

Frozen Section

A frozen section is a technique in which removed tissue is frozen, cut into thin slices, and stained for microscopic examination. A pathologist can rapidly complete a frozen section analysis, thus it is commonly used during surgery to quickly provide the surgeon with vital information such as a preliminary pathologic opinion of the presence or absence of prostate cancer (usually in the pelvic lymph nodes).

FSH
See Follicle-Stimulating Hormone.

G

Genadotropin-Releasing Hormone GNRH)
See LHRH Analogs and Luteinizing Hormone-Releasing Hormone.

Gastrointestinal
Gastrointestinal is related to the digestive system and/or the intestines.

Genetic Drift
As a cancer grows, it may go from a well-differentiated, slow-growing tumor to a poorly differentiated, aggressive malignancy. This process is called genetic drift.

Genital System
The genital system is the biological system that (in males) includes the testicles, vas deferens, prostate, and penis.

Genitourinary System
The genitourinary system is the combined genital and urinary systems; also known as the genitourinary tract.

Gland
A gland is a structure or organ that produces a substance used in another part of the body.

Gleason
Gleason is the name of a pathologist who developed the Gleason grading system commonly used to grade prostate cancer.

Gleason Grading System
The Gleason grading system is named after the pathologist who developed this system for grading the aggressiveness of a tumor by describing its physical characteristics. On a total scale of 2 to 10, the higher the grade, the more aggressive, or fast-growing, the cancer appears to be.

Gleason Score
A Gleason score is a widely used method for classifying the cellular differentiation of cancerous tissues; the less the cancerous cells appear like normal cells, the more malignant the cancer; two numbers, each from 1–5, are assigned successively to the two most predominant patterns of differentiation present in the examined tissue sample and are added together to produce the total Gleason score; high numbers indicate poor differentiation and therefore cancer.

Goserelin

Goserelin is the generic name for the antiandrogen drug Z®oladex, used to treat advanced prostate cancer.

Goserelin Acetate

Goserelin acetate is a luteinizing hormone-releasing hormone (LHRH) analog used in the palliative hormonal treatment of advanced prostate cancer and sometimes in the adjuvant and neoadjuvant hormonal treatment of earlier stages of prostate cancer.

Grade

Grade is a means of describing the potential degree of severity of a cancer based on the appearance of cancer cells under a microscope (see Gleason Score).

Growth Factors

Growth factors are molecules in the body that can increase the amount of cell division, or growth. Sometimes they can also stimulate cancer growth. Some of the most powerful chemotherapeutic drugs are believed to work by blocking growth factors that a cancer might need to survive.

Gynecomastia

Gynecomastia is the enlargement or tenderness of the male breasts or nipples; a possible side effect of hormonal therapy.

H

Hematospermia

Hematospermia is the occurrence of blood in the semen.

Hematuria

Hematuria is the occurrence of blood in the urine.

Heparin

See Anticoagulant.

Hereditary

Something inherited from one's parents and earlier generations is hereditary. It is the historical distribution of biological characteristics through a group of related individuals via their DNA.

Hereditary Prostate Cancer

Prostate cancer can be hereditary. A family has hereditary prostate cancer if:

▶ Three first-degree relatives (a father and at least two brothers) have had prostate cancer at any age.

▶ Two first-degree relatives (a father and one or more brothers) have had prostate cancer before the age of 55.

▶ Three generations of the family have had a father, grandfather or son with prostate cancer.

Hesitancy

Hesitancy is difficulty in starting urine flow.

High-Dose-Rate (HDR) Prostate Brachytherapy

High-dose-rate (HDR) prostate brachytherapy (also called temporary iridium template therapy) is a temporary radioactive seed implantation procedure. Radioactive iridium seeds are temporarily implanted in the prostate, followed by external-beam radiation therapy. The complication rate, time lost, pain, and dollar cost with the permanent seed implant procedure is lower than with this procedure, but it seems to have the same results with respect to the local control of cancer.

HIFU

See High-Intensity Focused Ultrasound.

High-Intensity Focused Ultrasound

High-intensity focused ultrasound (HIFU) is a treatment for benign prostatic enlargement that uses heat from ultrasound energy like a knife to trim excess prostate tissue that may cause urinary problems.

Histology

Histology is the study of the appearance and behavior of tissue, usually carried out under a microscope by a pathologist (who is a physician) or a histologist (who is not necessarily a physician).

Hormone

Hormones are biologically active chemicals that are responsible for many important body functions and the development of secondary sexual characteristics.

Hormone Therapy

Hormone therapy involves the use of hormones, hormone analogs, and certain surgical techniques to treat disease (in this case, advanced prostate cancer). The purpose of hormonal therapy in general is to lower testosterone to castrate or prepuberty levels. Hormones are used either on their own or in combination with other hormones or in combination with other methods of treatment; because prostate cancer is usually dependent on male hormones to grow, hormonal therapy can be an effective means of alleviating symptoms and retarding the development of the disease.

Hormone-Dependent vs. Hormone-Independent Prostate Cancer

Hormone-dependent cancer needs hormones from the body to grow and live. If someone has prostate cancer it is better to have the hormone-dependent variety, because today's treatments can shut off the hormone production that fuels cancer growth. Hormone-independent cells, on the other hand, can thrive without the presence of hormones—they will continue to grow regardless of whether the hormone supply is cut off. Therefore, some other type of treatment other than hormonal therapy (radiation, surgery or cryosurgery) is needed to try and stop these cells from growing.

Hormone-Deprivation Therapy
See Hormone Therapy.

Hot Flash
A hot flash is the sudden sensation of warmth in the face, neck, and upper body; a side effect of many forms of hormone therapy.

Hot Spots
Hot spots are images on a bone scan that indicate where prostate cancer has spread to the bones.

Hypercalcemia
Hypercalcemia is abnormally high concentrations of calcium in the blood, indicating leeching of calcium from bone (tumors raise serum calcium levels by destroying bone by releasing PTH or a PTH-like substance, osteoclast-activating factor, prostaglandins, and perhaps, a vitamin D-like sterol). Symptoms of hypercalcemia may include drowsiness, lethargy, headaches, depression or apathy, irritability, confusion, weakness, muscle flaccidity, bone pain, pathologic fractures, signs of heart block, cardiac arrest in systole, hypertension, anorexia, nausea, vomiting, constipation, dehydration, polydipsia, renal polyuria, flank pain, and eventually azotemia (excess of urea or other nitrogenous substances in the blood). Hypercalcemia is rare in prostate cancer.

Hyperplasia
Hyperplasia is the enlargement of an organ or tissue because of an increase in the number of cells in that organ or tissue. See also Benign Prostatic Hypertrophy.

Hyper-Reflexive
Hyper-reflexive usually refers to a spastic, or overactive, bladder, characterized by urgency (the strong desire to urinate) and urge incontinence (the strong urge that results in urine leakage).

Hyperthermia
Hyperthermia is treatment that uses heat. For example, heat produced by microwave radiation.

Hytrin®
See Alpha-Blockers.

I

Imaging
Imaging is a technique or method allowing a physician to see something that would not normally be visible. An X-ray, ultrasound, and ProstaScint® scan are all examples of imaging techniques.

Immune System
The immune system is the biological system that protects a person or animal from the effects of foreign materials such as bacteria, cancer cells, and other things, which might make that person or animal sick.

Implant

An implant is a device that is inserted into the body; e.g., a tiny container of radioactive material inserted in or near a tumor; also a device inserted in order to replace or substitute for an ability that has been lost. For example, a penile implant is a device that can be surgically inserted into the penis to provide rigidity for intercourse.

Impotence

Impotence is the partial or total loss of an erection, which can be caused by a variety of prostate-cancer treatments or by older age. The condition may be temporary or permanent. Regardless of the cause, it can be treated by medication, a vacuum device or the injection of a drug into the penis to increase blood flow to the organ.

Incidental

Incidental is something that is insignificant or irrelevant. For example, incidental prostate cancer (also known as latent prostate cancer) is a form of prostate cancer that is of no clinical significance to the person in whom it is discovered.

Incision

An incision is a cut made by a surgeon to get to the structure to be fixed or removed.

Incontinence

Incontinence (urinary incontinence) is the loss of urinary control. There are various kinds and degrees of incontinence; overflow incontinence is a condition in which the bladder retains urine after voiding; as a consequence, the bladder remains full most of the time, resulting in involuntary seepage of urine from the bladder; stress incontinence is the involuntary discharge of urine when there is increased pressure upon the bladder, as in coughing or straining to lift heavy objects; total incontinence is the inability to voluntarily exercise control over the sphincters of the bladder neck and urethra, resulting in total loss of retentive ability.

Indication

An indication is a reason for doing something or taking some action; also used to mean the approved clinical application of a drug.

Infectious Prostatitis

Infectious prostatitis is also called chronic or acute bacterial prostatitis, a type of inflammation of the prostate.

Inflammation

An inflammation is any form of swelling or pain or irritation.

Informed Consent

Informed consent is permission to proceed given by someone after being fully informed of the purposes and potential consequences of a medical procedure.

Insulin-like Growth Factor (IGF)
A circulating hormone that helps prostate cancer cells to grow. The level in the blood may be a risk factor for developing prostate cancer.

Interferon
Interferon is a body protein that affects antibody production and can modulate (regulate) the immune system.

Intermittent Androgen Blockade (IAB)
A type of hormonal therapy in which hormone therapy is cycled on and off over a period of months to try and decrease the side-effects of hormonal therapy.

Interstitial
Interstitial is within a particular organ. For example, interstitial prostate radiation therapy is radiation therapy applied within the prostate using implanted radioactive pellets or seeds. See also Brachytherapy.

Intravenous
Intravenous is the delivery of fluids and nutritional supplements into the body through a vein, usually in the arm, also called an "IV."

Intravenous Pyelogram (IVP)
An intravenous pyelogram (IVP) is a procedure that introduces an X-ray absorbing dye into the urinary tract in order to allow the physician a superior image of the tract by taking an X-ray. This test is rarely used to check for the spread of cancer to the kidneys and bladder but is a common test done for other conditions besides prostate cancer.

Invasive
An invasive procedure requires an incision or the insertion of an instrument or substance into the body.

Investigational Treatment
An investigational treatment or device is one that has not been approved by the FDA. This does not mean it is ineffective or unsafe, just that there has not been enough data collected to make a solid decision regarding its approval.

IV
See Intravenous.

K

Kegel Exercises
Kegel exercises are exercises designed to improve the strength of the muscles used in urinating.

Ketoconazole (Nizoral®)
Ketoconazole (Nizoral®) is a drug that can be used as a second-line hormonal agent when primary castration therapy fails.

Kidney

The kidney is one of a pair of organs whose primary function is to filter the fluids passing through the body.

L

Laparoscopy

Laparoscopy is a procedure that involves making a small abdominal incision through which a viewing tube is placed. It allows the doctor to look at the lymph nodes near the prostate and to biopsy them with long, thin surgical instruments. This procedure can help with the staging of prostate cancer. It is also used to observe the inside of the abdomen.

Latent

Latent is insignificant or irrelevant. For example, latent prostate cancer (also known as incidental prostate cancer) is a form of prostate cancer that is of no clinical significance.

Lateral-Lobe Enlargement

Lateral-lobe enlargement is a type of benign prostatic hyperplasia, or enlargement, in which prostate tissue squeezes the sides of the urethra and thus can cause urinary problems.

Leuprolide

Leuprolide is the generic name for the prostate-cancer drug n®,upron, which shuts of the production of testosterone.

Leuprolide Acetate

Leuprolide acetate is an LHRH analog.

LHRH

See Luteinizing Hormone-Releasing Hormone.

LHRH Analogs (or Agonists)

LHRH analogs (or agonists) are synthetic compounds that are chemically similar to luteinizing hormone-releasing hormone (LHRH), but are sufficiently different. They suppress testicular production of testosterone by binding to the LHRH receptor in the pituitary gland and either have no biological activity and therefore competitively inhibit the action of LHRH, or have LHRH activity that exhausts the production of LH by the pituitary. They are used in the palliative hormonal treatment of advanced prostate cancer and sometimes in the adjuvant and neoadjuvant hormonal treatment of earlier stages of prostate cancer.

Libido

Libido is an interest in sexual activity.

LNCap

LNCap is a line of human prostate cancer cells used in laboratory studies. This cell line is hormonally dependent.

Lobe
A lobe is one of the two sides of an organ that clearly has two sides (e.g., the prostate or the brain).

Localized
Localized means restricted to a well-defined area.

Localized Prostate Cancer
Localized prostate cancer is cancer that is confined to the prostate gland.

Lupron®
Lupron® is the trade or brand name of Leuprolide Acetate, an LHRH agonist.

Luteinizing Hormone (LH)
Lutenizing hormone (LH) is a brain hormone that stimulates testosterone production in the testicles.

Luteinizing Hormone-Releasing Hormone (LHRH)
Luteinizing hormone-releasing hormone (LHRH) is the hormone responsible for stimulating the production of testosterone in the body.

Lymph (also Lymphatic Fluid)
Lymph (also lymphatic fluid) is the clear fluid in which all of the cells in the body are constantly bathed; carries cells that help fight infection.

Lymphadenectomy
Lymphadenectomy (also known as a pelvic lymph node dissection) is a procedure that involves the removal and microscopic examination of selected lymph nodes, a common site of metastatic disease with prostate cancer. This procedure can be performed during surgery prior to the removal of the prostate gland, or by means of a small incision, a "laparoscopic lymphadenectomy" may be performed, a simple operation requiring only an overnight hospital stay.

Lymphatic System
The lymphatic system is the tissue and organs that produce, store, and carry cells that fight infection; includes bone marrow, spleen, thymus, lymph nodes, and channels that carry lymph fluid.

Lymph Nodes
Lymph nodes are the small glands that occur throughout the body and which filter the clear fluid known as lymph or lymphatic fluid. Lymph nodes filter out bacteria and other toxins, as well as cancer cells.

Lymph-Node Dissection
See Lymphadenectomy.

M

MAB
Maximal Androgen Blockade (see CHT, CHB, ADT).

MAD
Maximal Androgen Deprivation (see ADT, CHB, CHT).

Magnetic Resonance
Magnetic resonance is the absorption of specific frequencies of radio and microwave radiation by atoms placed in a strong magnetic field.

Magnetic Resonance Imaging (MRI)
Magnetic resonance imaging (MRI) is the use of magnetic resonance with atoms in body tissues to produce distinct cross-sectional, and even three-dimensional images of internal organs. MRI is primarily of use in staging biopsy-proven prostate cancer.

Malignancy
A malignancy is a growth or tumor composed of cancerous cells.

Malignant
Malignant or cancerous; tending to become progressively worse and to result in death; having the invasive and metastatic (spreading) properties of cancer.

Margin
Margin is normally used to mean the "surgical margin," which is the outer edge of the tissue removed during surgery; if the surgical margin shows no sign of cancer ("negative margins"), the prognosis for cure is generally better than if the margins are positive.

Margin of the Prostate
Margin of the prostate refers to the outside surface of the prostate gland. If cancer has invaded the margin it is called "margin positive" and if it has not invaded this area it is called "margin negative."

Maximal Androgen Blockade
See Combined Androgen Deprivation Therapy.

Medical Oncologist
A medical oncologist is an oncologist primarily trained in the use of medicines (rather than surgery) to treat cancer.

Megesterol Acetate
Megesterol acetate (Megace) is a drug used to stimulate appetite.

Metastasis
(the plural form is metastases)
Metastasis is the spread of cancer beyond its primary location to other sites in the body such as the bones, lungs, bloodstream, or other nearby structures.

Metastasize
Metastasize is the spread of a malignant tumor to other parts of the body.

Metastatic
Metastatic is having the characteristics of a secondary tumor.

Metastatic Workup

A metastatic workup is a group of tests, including bone scans, X-rays, and blood tests, to determine whether cancer has metastasized.

Metastron®

Metastron® is the brand or trade name of Strontium-89 in the United States.

Microtubules

Microtubule are scaffold-like structures in a cell that control cell division. Many chemotherapy drugs target the microtubules.

Middle-Lobe Enlargement

Middle-lobe enlargement is a form of benign prostatic hyperplasia (BPH) in which part of the prostate grows up into the bladder. This tissue can partially or totally block the drainage of urine from the bladder into the urethra.

Minilap

See Mini-Laparotomy.

Mini-Laparotomy

A mini-laparotomy (also called a "minilap" or a "staging pelvic lymphadenectomy") is a procedure in which a small incision is made, through which the pelvic lymph nodes are examined. If they are not cancerous, the incision is enlarged and the prostate is surgically removed. If the nodes are found to have cancer, the incision is closed and other treatment options are considered.

Mis-staging

Mis-staging is the assignment of an incorrect clinical stage at initial diagnosis because of the difficulty of assessing the available information with accuracy.

Mitosis

Mitosis is the process of a cell dividing into two cells. This is controlled by the microtubules (see Microtubules).

Mitoxantrone (Novantrone®)

Mitoxantrone (Novantrone®) is a chemotherapy drug for prostate cancer that has been shown to decrease pain when used in conjunction with prednisone (a steroid medicine). It is approved for this use in prostate cancer by the FDA.

Moderately Differentiated

See Differentiation of Prostate Cancer Cells.

Monoclonal

Monoclonal means formed from a single group of identical cells. It can also refer to antibodies that only react to a single type of antigen.

Morbidity

Morbidity is unhealthy consequences and complications resulting from treatment.

Monotherapy
See Single-Agent Androgen Deprivation Therapy.

MRI
See Magnetic Resonance Imaging.

N

National Cancer Institute
The National Cancer Institute (NCI) is an arm of the National Institutes of Health (NIH) located in Bethesda, MD. The NCI organizes and funds many clinical research trials and helps establish guidelines for cancer treatment and research in the United States.

NCI
See National Cancer Institute.

Negative
Negative is the term used to describe a test result that does not show the presence of the substance or material for which the test was carried out. For example, a negative bone scan would show no sign of bone metastases.

Neoadjuvant Hormone Therapy
Neoadjuvant hormone therapy is the use of hormonal therapy to shrink or contain the prostate cancer prior to radical prostatectomy (surgical removal of the prostate) or radiation therapy.

Neoplasia
Neoplasia is the growth of cells under conditions that would tend to prevent the development of normal tissue (e.g., a cancer).

Nerve Sparing
Nerve sparing is the term used to describe a type of prostatectomy in which the surgeon saves the nerves that affect sexual and related functions.

Nerve-Sparing Radical Prostatectomy
Nerve-sparing radical prostatectomy is an operation to remove the prostate that allows at least one of the two nerve bundles near the gland to be saved. Sparing these nerves greatly increases a man's chance of retaining normal sexual function.

Neuron-specific Enolase
Neuron-specific enolase (NSE) is a neuroendocrine marker (see CGA).

Neurovascular Bundles
Neurovascular bundles are two bundles of nerves and blood vessels, one located on each side of the prostate, that help a man achieve an erection. Removal of or injury to both nerve bundles results in impotence. Sparing at least one of these bundles in most cases allows a man to keep having normal erections.

NIH (National Institutes of Health)
See National Cancer Institute.

Nilandron®

Nilandron® is an antiandrogen that is used in the treatment of prostate cancer. Made by Hoechst Marion Roussel, it is also known by the generic name nilutamide.

Nilutamide

Nilutamide is an antiandrogen. Also see Nilandron®.

Nocturia

Nocturia is waking up many times in the night to urinate, a common symptom of benign prostatic hyperplasia (BPH).

Nonbacterial Prostatitis

Nonbacterial prostatitis is inflammation of the prostate, the cause of which is unknown. Symptoms include painful, difficult urination and pain in the penis, scrotum, perineum, lower back, and general pubic area.

Noninvasive

A medical test or procedure that does not require an incision or insertion of an instrument or substance into the body is considered to be noninvasive.

NSE

See Neuron-specific Enolase.

Nuclear Medicine

Nuclear medicine is the department in the hospital where bone scans are usually performed. Bone scans help the doctor to determine whether a man's prostate cancer has spread into the skeleton.

ng/ml

The abbreviation for nanogram per milliliter is ng/ml. A nanogram is one-billionth of a gram, and a milliliter is one-thousandth of a liter. Whenever a man gets a PSA test, the result is reported in ng/ml. For example, a PSA test result of 3 actually means 3 ng/ml. The larger the number, the higher the level of PSA in the bloodstream.

O

Oncologist

An oncologist is a physician who specializes in the treatment of various types of cancer.

Oncology

Oncology is the branch of medical science dealing with tumors; an oncologist is a specialist in the study of cancerous tumors.

Orchiectomy

Orchiectomy is the surgical removal of the testicles.

Organ

An organ is a group of tissues that work in concert to carry out a specific set of functions (e.g., the heart, lungs, or prostate).

Organ-Confined

Organ-confined refers to cancer that is still entirely located within the organ or gland in which it started.

Orgasm

An orgasm is sexual climax, characterized by ejaculation in men.

Osteoblast

An osteoblast is a cell that forms bone.

Osteoclast

An osteoc last is a cell that breaks down a bone cell, grows in bone tissue, and apparently absorbs bone tissue.

Osteolysis

Osteolysis is the destruction of bone.

Osteopenia

Low bone density

Osteoporosis

Low bone density that is usually treated with medicines such as bisphosphonates.

Overflow Incontinence

Overflow incontinence is urine leakage caused by a full bladder.

Overstaging

Overstaging is the assignment of an overly high clinical stage at initial diagnosis because of the difficulty of assessing the available information with accuracy (e.g., stage T3b as opposed to stage T2b).

P

Paclitaxel (Taxol®)

Paclitaxel (Taxol®) is a commonly used chemotherapy agent for hormone-refractory prostate cancer. It is a microtubule inhibitor. It is often used with estramustine.

Palliative Treatment

Palliative treatment is designed to relieve a particular problem without necessarily solving it. For example, palliative therapy is given in order to relieve symptoms and improve quality of life, but does not provide a cure.

Palpable

Palpable is something that is capable of being felt during a physical examination by an experienced physician; in the case of prostate cancer, this normally refers to some form of abnormality of the prostate that can be felt during a digital rectal examination.

PAP

See Prostatic Acid Phosphatase.

Pathologist

A pathologist is a doctor who examines the tissues and cells of the body under a microscope to determine what type of disease is present. A pathologist will assign a Gleason score to the prostate cancer and also help stage the disease. A pathologist specializing in urological problems such as prostate cancer is called a uro-pathologist.

Pathological Staging of Prostate Cancer

Pathological staging of prostate cancer is the evaluation of the prostate tissue removed during surgery to determine how far the cancer has spread.

PCa

See prostate cancer

PDQ

See Physicians Data Query (PDQ).

Pelvis

The pelvis is that part of the skeleton that joins the lower limbs of the body together.

Pelvic Area

The pelvic area is the area of the body below the waist, including the genital region.

Penile

Penile refers to anything related to the penis. For example, penile implants help to make the penis erect.

Penile Implants

Penile implants are mechanical, inflatable, and bendable devices that, once surgically inserted into the penis, help with erectile dysfunction and impotence.

Penis

The penis the male organ used in urination and intercourse.

Perineal

Relating to the perineum.

Perineural Invasion

Invasion into the nerves of the prostate by the cancer. This is usually a sign of a more aggressive cancer.

Perineum

The perineum is the area of the body between the scrotum and the rectum; a perineal procedure utilizes this area as the point of entry to the body.

Peripheral

Peripheral is outside the central region.

Peripheral Zone (PZ)

The peripheral zone (PZ) of the prostate is the largest part of the prostate, where about 70% of all prostate cancers begin to grow. This is also the only area of the gland that can be felt during a digital rectal exam.

Periprostatic Tissue

Periprostatic tissue is the tissue just outside the prostate. If cancer has spread to the periprostatic tissue, then it is no longer localized, or confined.

Periurethral Zone

The periurethral zone is the smallest zone of the prostate, which surrounds the urethra. Cancer rarely begins growing in this area.

PET Scan

See Positron Emission Tomography.

Phenotype

How something looks to the eye.

Physicians Data Query (PDQ)

Physicians Data Query (PDQ) is a NCI supported database available to physicians, containing current information on standard treatments and ongoing clinical trials.

PIN

See Prostatic Intraepithelial (or Intraductal) Neoplasia) (PIN).

Placebo

A placebo is a pill or other substance that contains no real medicine. In some studies, placebos are given to one group of unsuspecting people while another group unknowingly receives a real drug. The reactions of the two groups are then compared to test the effectiveness of the real medication.

Placebo Effect

Placebo effect is a commonly observed phenomenon in which people receiving a placebo actually have some improvement in their symptoms, even though the pill or substance they have been taking contains no real medicine.

Polyploid

Polyploid refers to an extra set of chromosomes, which could indicate an abnormal or cancerous cell. Recent blood tests (flow cytometry, static image analysis) can detect polyploid cells in the bloodstream, which could indicate that a cancer has grown beyond the prostate.

Ploidy

Ploidy is a term used to describe the number of sets of chromosomes in a cell (see also Diploid and Aneuploid).

Poorly Differentiated

See Differentiation.

Positive

Positive is the term used to describe a test result that shows the presence of the substance or material for which the test was carried out. For example, a positive bone scan would show signs of bone metastases.

Positron Emission Tomography (PET)

Positron emission tomography (PET) uses a radioactive isotope that is taken up by tumor tissue to show that the tumor is functional. Current studies do not indicate a high utility of PET scanning in prostate cancer that is newly diagnosed, perhaps related to the usual slow doubling times.

Posterior

Posterior or the rear; for example, the posterior of the prostate faces a man's back

Prednisone

Prednisone is a steroid medicine that is often used in advanced prostate cancer as a single agent or in combination with other medicines.

Proctitis

Proctitis is an inflammation of the rectum. This can be a side effect of radiation therapy, but it usually lasts for a short time. Symptoms include rectal bleeding, pain, and diarrhea.

Prognosis

A prognosis is an estimation of how good or bad someone will do in the future based on all of the available medical information, including the treatment the person is currently undergoing.

Progression

Progression is the continuing growth or regrowth of the cancer.

Progression-free

This refers to the length of time that cancer cannot be detected after it is treated.

Prolactin (PRL)

Prolactin (PRL) is a trophic hormone produced by the pituitary that increases androgen receptors, increases sensitivity to androgens, and regulates production and secretion of citrate.

Proscar®

Proscar® is the brand name of finasteride.

ProstaScint®

ProstaScint® is a monoclonal antibody test directed against the prostate-specific membrane antigen (PSMA). It seems to focus on androgen-independent tumor tissue.

Prostate

The prostate is a muscular, walnut-shaped gland located below the bladder and above the rectum in males. The prostate produces about a third of the fluid that makes up semen. This fluid nourishes the sperm and helps them survive inside the woman's body so pregnancy has a better chance of occurring.

Prostate Cancer

Cancer that starts in the prostate gland.

Prostatectomy

Prostatectomy is the surgical removal of part or all of the prostate gland.

Prostate-Specific Antigen (PSA)

PSA (prostate-specific antigen) is a protein secreted by the epithelial cells of the prostate gland including cancer cells that leaks into the blood. An elevated level in the blood indicates an abnormal condition of the prostate gland, either benign or malignant. An annual prostate checkup should include both a PSA blood test and a digital rectal exam (see Screening).

Prostate-Specific Membrane Antigen (PSMA)

Prostate-specific membrane antigen (PSMA) is a protein that is found on the membranes of prostate cells. This antibody forms the basis of the ProstaScint® test (see Monoclonal).

Prostatic Acid Phosphatase (PAP)

Prostatic acid phosphatase (PAP) is an enzyme now measured only rarely to decide whether prostate cancer has escaped from the prostate.

Prostatic Intraepithelial (or Intraductal) Neoplasia) (PIN)

Prostatic intraepithelial (or intraductal) neoplasia) (PIN) is a pathologically identifiable condition believed to be a possible precursor of prostate cancer, also known more simply as dysplasia by many physicians.

Prostatitis

Prostatitis is an infection or inflammation of the prostate gland treatable by medication and/or manipulation. BPH is a more permanent laying down of fibroblasts and connective tissue caused when the prostate tries to contain a relatively silent chronic lower-grade infection, often requiring a TURP to relieve the symptoms.

Prosthesis

Prosthesis is a man-made device used to replace a normal body part or function.

Protocol

A protocol is a precise set of methods by which a research study is to be carried out.

PSA (Prostate-Specific Antigen)

See Prostate-Specific Antigen (PSA).

PSA (free)

A free PSA assay, reports the percentage of free-PSA to total-PSA (total PSA = free PSA + bound PSA). It is helpful for screening purposes when PSA values are above the normal threshold for an age group(greater than 4), but less than 10. One study showed that men with PSA ratio >25% had no PCa; those with <10% were likely to have PCa. This test is not yet available everywhere.

PSA Density

PSA density is a formula used to determine a man's chances of having prostate cancer and thus the need for a biopsy. It involves dividing the PSA value (in ng/ml) by the volume, or size, of the prostate (based on transrectal ultrasound).

PSA RT-PCR

See PSA Reverse Transcriptase, Polymerase Chain Reaction (PSA RT-PCR).

PSA Reverse Transcriptase Polymerase Chain Reaction (PSA RT-PCR)

PSA reverse transcriptase polymerase chain reaction (PSA RT-PCR) is a blood test that detects micrometastatic cells circulating in the bloodstream. The test may be useful as a screening tool to help avoid unnecessary invasive treatments (RP, RT etc.) for men with metastasized PCa. It is still considered experimental and is not routinely offered.

PSA Velocity

PSA velocity is the change in PSA level over time. The currently accepted normal annual PSA increase is 0.75 ng/ml. PSA velocity is particularly useful in monitoring two types of men: those whose PSA level is increasing rapidly but is still within the normal range, and those with a suspiciously high PSA level who have normal biopsy results.

PZ

See Peripheral Zone (PZ).

Q

Quality of Life

Quality of life is an evaluation of health status relative to someone's age, expectations, and physical and mental capabilities.

R

Radiation Oncologist

A radiation oncologist is a physician who has received special training regarding the treatment of cancers with different types of radiation.

Radiation Therapy (RT)

Radiation therapy is a general term to describe radiation treatment. However, radiation treatment can come from an outside source (external-beam radiation therapy) or it can come from an internal source (radioactive seed implants).

Radical

Radical (in a surgical sense) refers to something directed at the cause of a disease. Thus, radical prostatectomy is the surgical removal of the prostate with the intent to cure the problem believed to be caused by or within the prostate.

Radical Prostatectomy

Radical prostatectomy is the surgical removal of the prostate. There are two types of radical prostatectomy: "retropubic," in which an incision is made in the abdomen; and "perineal," in which an incision is made between the scrotum and anus.

Radioactive-Seed Implantation

See Brachytherapy.

Radioactive Scintigraphy
See Bone Scan.

Radioisotope
A radioisotope is a type of atom (or a chemical that is made with a type of atom) that emits radioactivity.

Radio Sensitivity
Radio sensitivity is the degree to which a type of cancer responds to radiation therapy.

Radiotherapy
Radiotherapy refers to treatment with radiation.

Randomized
Randomized is the process of assigning individuals to different forms of treatment in a research study in a random manner.

Rectal Exam
See Digital Rectal Exam.

Rectum
The rectum is the lower part of the small intestine that ends at the anus.

Recurrence
Recurrence is when cancer returns after initial treatment.

Refractory
Refractory is resistance to therapy. For example, hormone-refractory prostate cancer is resistant to forms of treatment based on the use of hormones.

Regression
Regression is a reduction in the size of a single tumor or reduction in the number and/or size of several tumors.

Remission
Remission is the real or apparent disappearance of some or all of the signs or symptoms of cancer; the period (temporary or permanent) during which a disease remains under control, without progressing; even complete remission does not necessarily indicate cure.

Resection
Resection is surgical removal.

Resectoscope
A resectoscope is an instrument inserted through the urethra to remove tissue (usually from the prostate).

Resistance
Resistance (in the medical sense) is someone's ability to fight off a disease as a result of the effectiveness of their immune system.

Response
A response is a decrease in disease that occurs because of treatment.

Retention

Retention is the difficulty in initiation of urination or the inability to completely empty the bladder.

Retropubic Prostatectomy

Retropubic prostatectomy is the surgical removal of the prostate through an incision in the abdomen.

Retrograde Ejaculation

See Dry Ejaculation.

Reverse Transcriptase, Polymerase Chain Reaction (RT-PCR)

Reverse transcriptase, polymerase chain reaction (RT-PCR) is a technique that allows a physician to search for tiny quantities of protein, such as PSA, in the blood or other fluids and tissues (see Prostate-Specific Antigen (PSA).

Risk

Risk is the chance or probability that a particular event will or will not happen.

Risk Factor

A risk factor is something that increases a person's chances of getting a disease, such as cancer. For example, a high-fat and low-fiber diet may increase an individual's chance of getting prostate cancer.

RP

See Radical Prostatectomy.

RTCPR

See RT-PCR.

RT-PCR

See Reverse Transcriptase, Polymerase Chain Reaction.

S

Salvage

Salvage is a procedure intended to "rescue" someone following the failure of a prior treatment. For example, a salvage prostatectomy would be the surgical removal of the prostate after the failure of prior radiation therapy or cryosurgery

Salvage Therapy

Salvage therapy is a term used to describe a situation where the first line of treatment did not work and now another type of treatment is being tried. For example, if a radical prostatectomy is not successful, external-beam radiation treatment may then be used.

Sandwich Approach

A sandwich approach is when someone is given a week off about halfway through external-beam radiation therapy. This gives the bowel and bladder a chance to recover from the shock of treatment.

Screening

Screening is used to separate people with

tumors from those without tumors; multiple criteria are often used. The following PSA screening "cutoff" levels for PCa are replacing the older 4.0 value:

Age PSA Cutoff
40–49 up to 2.5
50–59 up to 3.5
60–69 up to 4.5
70–79 up to 6.5

Scrotum

The scrotum is the pouch of skin containing a man's testicles.

Secondary To

Secondary to is something derived from or consequent to a primary event or thing.

Selenium

Selenium is a relatively rare nonmetallic element found in food in small quantities, which may have some effect in prevention of cancer.

Sequential Androgen Blockade (SAB)

A type of hormonal therapy that uses finasteride and an nonsteroidal anti-androgen.

Semen

Semen is the part of the ejaculate (produced during male orgasm) that contains fluid and sperm. The sperm comes from the testicles and the fluid comes mostly from the prostate and the seminal vesicles.

Seminal

Seminal is related to the semen. For example, the seminal vesicles are glands at the base of the bladder and connected to the prostate that provide nutrients for the semen.

Seminal Vesicle

A seminal vesicle is a reproductive organ that is located close to the urethra and contributes about two-thirds of the fluid for semen. It is also a neighbor to the prostate and a place where prostate cancer may spread.

Sensitivity

Sensitivity is the probability that a diagnostic test can correctly identify the presence of a particular disease assuming the proper conduct of the test; specifically, the number of true positive results divided by the sum of the true positive results and the false negative results (see Specificity).

Sex Hormone-binding Globulin (SHBG)

A protein that binds testosterone in the blood.

Sextant

Sextant is something that has six parts. Thus, a sextant biopsy is a biopsy that takes six samples.

Sextant Biopsy

See Biopsy.

Side Effect

A side effect is a reaction to a medication or treatment (most commonly used to mean an unnecessary or undesirable effect).

Sign

A sign is a physical change that can be observed as a consequence of an illness or disease.

Sildenafil

See Viagra®

Single-Agent Androgen-Deprivation Therapy

Single-agent androgen-deprivation therapy is when a bilateral orchiectomy or LHRH agonist is used to interfere with the cancer cell's ability to interact with testosterone. This appears to be almost or just as effective as combined hormonal therapy for advanced prostate cancer.

Specificity

Specificity is the probability that a diagnostic test can correctly identify the absence of a particular disease assuming the proper conduct of the test. Specifically, it is the number of true negative results divided by the sum of the true negative results and the false positive results; a method that detects 95% of true PCa cases is highly sensitive, but if it also falsely indicates that 40% of those who do not have PCa do have PCa, then its specificity is 60%; rather poor.

Sphincter

A sphincter is muscle tissue that helps to open or close a body opening. For example, when the bladder sphincter opens, urine flows down into the urethra; when it closes, the bladder fills with urine.

Spinal Cord

The spinal cord is the group of nerves that runs down the middle of the back. These are protected by back bones (vertebral bodies).

Spinal Cord Compression

Spinal cord compression occurs when prostate cancer spreads to the spine and invades the spinal cord. This usually results in pain or tingling shooting down the legs. This is a medical emergency and the person should go to an emergency room immediately.

Spine

The spine is all of the backbones.

Spot Radiation

Spot radiation is external-beam radiation treatment for bone pain that is associated with advanced prostate cancer. Radiation targeted to painful areas of bone does not stop the cancer from growing, but it can help ease some of the pain.

Stage

Stage is a term used to define the size and physical extent of a cancer.

Staging

Staging is the process of assigning a cancer stage in an individual in light of all the available information. It is used to help determine appropriate therapy. There are two staging methods: the Whitmore-Jewett staging classification (1956) and the more detailed TNM (Tumor, Nodes, Metastases) classification (1998) of the American Joint Committee on Cancer and the International Union Against Cancer. Staging should be subcategorized as clinical staging and pathologic staging. Pathologic stage usually relates to what is found at the time of surgery. (Whitmore-Jewett) (TNM)

Stage A becomes T1

Stage B becomes T2

Stage C becomes T3

Whitmore-Jewett Stages

Stage A is a clinically undetectable tumor confined to the gland and is an incidental finding at the time of prostate surgery.

A1 Well-differentiated with focal involvement.

A2 Moderately or poorly differentiated or involves multiple foci in the gland.

Stage B is a tumor confined to the prostate gland.

B0 Nonpalpable, PSA-detected.

B1 Single nodule in one lobe of the prostate.

B2 More extensive involvement of one lobe or involvement of both lobes.

Stage C is a tumor clinically localized to the periprostatic area but extending through the prostatic capsule; seminal vesicles may be involved.

C1 Clinical extracapsular extension.

C2 Extracapsular tumor producing bladder outlet or ureteral obstruction.

Stage D is metastatic disease.

D0 Clinically localized disease (prostate only) but persistently elevated enzymatic serum acid phosphatase.

D1 Regional lymph nodes only.

D2 Distant lymph nodes, metastases to bone or visceral organs.

D3 Men with D2 prostate cancer who relapse after adequate endocrine therapy.

TNM Stages

T Primary Tumor

TX Primary tumor cannot be assessed.

T0 No evidence of primary tumor.

T1 Clinically nonapparent tumor not palpable or visible by imaging.

T1a Tumor incidental histologic finding in 5% or less of tissue resected.

T1b Tumor incidental histologic finding in more 5 % of tissue resected.

T1c Tumor identified by needle biopsy (e.g., because of elevated PSA).

T2 Tumor confined within the prostate.

T2a Tumor involves half of a lobe or less.

T2b Tumor involves more than half a lobe, but not both lobes.

T2c Tumor involves both lobes.

T3 Tumor extends through the prostatic capsule.

T3a Unilateral extracapsular extension.

T3b Bilateral extracapsular extension.

T3c Tumor invades the seminal vesicle(s).

T4 Tumor is fixed or invades adjacent structures other than the seminal vesicles.

T4a Tumor invades any of bladder neck, sphincter, or rectum.

T4b Tumor invades levator muscles and/or is fixed to the pelvic wall.

Regional Lymph Nodes (N)

NX Regional lymph nodes cannot be assessed.

N0 No regional lymph node metastasis.

N1 Metastasis in a single lymph node, 2 cm or less in greatest dimension.

N2 Metastasis in a single lymph node, more than 2 cm but not more than 5 cm in greatest dimension; or multiple lymph node metastases, none more than 5 cm in greatest dimension.

N3 Metastases in a lymph node more than 5 cm in greatest dimension.

Distant Metastases (M)

MX Presence of distant metastasis cannot be assessed.

M0 No distant metastasis.

M1 Distant metastasis.

M1a Nonregional lymph node(s).

M1b Bone(s).

M1c Other site(s).

Staging Pelvic Lymphadenectomy
See Mini-Laparotomy.

Stent
A stent is a tube used by a surgeon to drain fluids.

Stress Incontinence
Stress incontinence is a type of urinary incontinence caused by normal activities such as walking, lifting, or playing tennis.

Stricture
Stricture is scarring as a result of a procedure or an injury that constricts the flow of urine through the urethra.

Strontium-89 (Metastron®)
Strontium-89 (Metastr®on) is an injectable

radioactive product that is used to relieve bone pain for some men with prostate cancer that no longer responds to hormones or appropriate forms of chemotherapy.

Subcapsular

Subcapsular refers to under the capsule. For example, a subcapsular orchiectomy is a form of castration in which the contents of each testicle is removed but the testicular capsules are then closed and remain in the scrotum.

Surgical Margins

Surgical margins refer to the outer margins, or edges, of a prostate gland that has been surgically removed. A pathologist will examine these edges to see if they are free of cancer. If they are cancer-free, then there is a good chance the cancer did not go beyond the prostate and all of it was removed. If the margins contain cancer, chances are the disease has spread beyond the prostate.

Suture

A suture is a surgical stitch used in the closure of a cut or incision.

Symptom

A symptom is a feeling, sensation, or experience associated with or resulting from a physical or mental disorder and noticeable by an individual.

Symptomatic

Symptomatic means a person is feeling the effects of a disease. For example, one of the many possible effects, or symptoms, of advanced prostate cancer is lower-back pain.

Systemic

Systemic is throughout the whole body.

T

Tamsulosin

See Alpha-Blockers.

Temporary Iridium Template Therapy

See High-Dose-Rate (HDR) Brachytherapy.

Terazosin

See Alpha-Blockers.

Testicles (Testes)

The testicles (testes) are part of the male genitals. They are located below the penis, inside the scrotum. They produce sperm and most of the body's testosterone.

Testis

A testis is one of two male reproductive glands located inside the scrotum, which are the primary sources of the male hormone testosterone.

Testosterone (T)

Testosterone (T) is the male hormone or androgen that comprises most of the androgens in a man's body. It is chiefly produced by the testicles. It may be produced in tissues from precursors such as androstenedione. It is essential to complete male sexual function and fertility.

Therapy

Therapy is the treatment of disease or disability.

Three-Dimensional Treatment Planning and Conformal Therapy

Three-dimensional treatment planning and conformal therapy is a type of external-beam radiation therapy that uses computerized images from a CT scan to help precisely conform the radiation beam to the shape of the tumor. This allows the delivery of the most powerful dose of radiation to the prostate while minimizing the risk of damage to surrounding structures.

TNM

Tumor, Nodes, Metastases (see Staging).

Total Androgen Blockade

See Combined Androgen-Deprivation Therapy.

Transition

Transition or change; for example, the transition zone of the prostate is the area of the prostate closest to the urethra and has features that distinguish it from the much larger peripheral zone.

Transition Zone (TZ)

The transition zone (TZ) is the innermost part of the prostate that surrounds the urethra as it leaves the bladder. This is where benign prostatic hyperplasia occurs, as well as a small percentage (15% to 20%) of prostate cancers.

Transperineal

Transperineal or through the perineum.

Transrectal

Transrectal refers to any procedure that is done through the rectum, such as ultrasound imaging and biopsy of the prostate.

Transrectal Ultrasound (TRUS)

Transrectal ultrasound (TRUS) is a diagnostic procedure that uses echoes of ultrasound waves (far beyond the hearing range) to image the prostate by inserting an ultrasound probe into the rectum; commonly used to visualize prostate biopsy procedures.

Transrectal Ultrasound (TRUS)-Guided Biopsy of the Prostate

Transrectal ultrasound (TRUS)-guided biopsy of the prostate is a prostate biopsy that is performed under the guidance of transrectal ultrasound, in which sound waves from a rectal ultrasound probe act as a navigator to let the doctor accurately locate the prostate for tissue sampling. A tiny needle is then inserted alongside the probe to remove a small sample of prostate tissue. Usually a minimum of six individual biopsies are taken from different areas of the prostate.

Transurethral
Transurethral is through the urethra.

**Transurethral Resection
    of the Prostate (TURP)**
Transurethral resection of the prostate (TURP) is a treatment for benign prostatic hyperplasia in which fragments of the enlarged prostate are removed to help improve urine flow. TURP is performed through a catheter inserted into the penis, so there is no incision involved.

**Treatment-Planning CT Scan
    of the Prostate**
A treatment-planning CT scan of the prostate involves using a CT scan to get a better understanding of the exact position of the prostate. This helps plan the most effective way to deliver radiation during treatment.

Treatment
Treatment is the administration of remedies to someone for a disease.

TRUS
See Transrectal Ultrasound (TRUS).

TRUS-P
See TRUS.

Tumor
A tumor is an excessive growth of cells caused by uncontrolled and disorderly cell replacement; an abnormal tissue growth that can be either benign or malignant (see Benign, Malignant).

TURP
See Transurethral Resection of the Prostate (TURP).

TUR/P
See TURP.

TZ
See Transition Zone (TZ).

U

Ultrasound
An ultrasound uses sound waves at a particular frequency (far beyond the hearing range) whose echoes bouncing off tissue can be used to image internal organs (e.g., a baby in the uterus).

Understaging
Understaging is the assignment of an overly low clinical stage at initial diagnosis because

of the difficulty of assessing the available information with accuracy (e.g., stage T2b as opposed to stage T3b).

Unit

A unit is a surgical term for a pint (usually of blood).

Ureter

The ureter is an anatomical tube that drains urine from one of the two kidneys to the bladder.

Urethra

The urethra is the tube that drains urine from the bladder through the prostate and out through the penis.

Urethral Sphincter

The urethral sphincter is the muscle located just below the penis which, along with the bladder neck, is responsible for urinary control.

Urethral Stricture

Urethral stricture is the scarring and narrowing of the urethra, often a complication of surgical treatment for prostate disease.

Urgency

Urgency is the feeling of immediately having to urinate.

Urinary Incontinence

Urinary incontinence is the loss of some or all urinary control, resulting in the leakage of urine from the bladder.

Urinary Retention

Urinary retention is when the bladder cannot empty and remains completely or partially full.

Urinary System

The urinary system is the group of organs and their interconnections that permits excess, filtered fluids to exit the body, including (in the male) the kidneys, the ureters, bladder, urethra, and penis.

Urologist

A urologist is a doctor trained first as a surgeon who specializes in disorders of the genitourinary system.

Urinary Tract Infection (UTI)

A urinary tract infection (UTI) is an infection identifiable by the presence of bacteria (or theoretically, viruses) in the urine. It may be associated with a fever or a burning sensation on urination.

UTI

See Urinary Tract Infection (UTI).

V

Vas Deferens

The vas deferens is the tube through which sperm travels from the testes to the prostate prior to ejaculation.

Vacuum-Erection Device

A vacuum-erection device is a medical device used to create an erection. It is used by men who can no longer achieve an erection naturally. It consists of a tube that is placed over the penis, through which a vacuum is created that draws blood into the organ. The tube is then removed and a ring is placed at the base of the penis to keep the erection from subsiding. The ring can be left in place for up to 30 minutes.

Vasectomy

A vasectomy is an operation to make a man sterile by cutting the vas deferens, thus preventing passage of sperm from the testes to the prostate.

Vertebral Bodies

Vertebral bodies are the individual backbones. They hold an individual erect and protect the spinal cord.

Vesicle

A vesicle is a small sac containing a biologically important fluid.

Viagra®

A medicine used to help men with erection difficulties. The trade name for the drug sildenafil.

Vinblastine (Velban®)

Vinblastine (Velban®) is a chemotherapy agent that attacks the microtubules. Often used with estramustine.

W

Watchful Waiting

Watchful waiting is when a man diagnosed with prostate cancer decides to carefully monitor the progress of his cancer rather than opting for immediate treatment. This is an active process that involves the man and his doctor.

Well-Differentiated Prostate Cancer

See Differentiation.

Whitmore-Jewett Staging

See Staging.

X

X-Ray

An X-ray is a type of high energy radiation that can be used at low levels to make images of the internal structures of the body and at high levels for radiation therapy.

Z

Zoladex®

Zoladex® is the trade or brand name for goserelin acetate, a LHRH agonist.

Zone

A zone is a part or area of an organ.

Index

Index

D

E

APPOINTMENTS

Date
Doctor
Location
Telephone
Questions

Comments

Date
Doctor
Location
Telephone
Questions

Comments

APPOINTMENTS

Date _____

Doctor _____

Location _____

Telephone _____

Questions _____

_____

Comments _____

_____

_____

Date _____

Doctor _____

Location _____

Telephone _____

Questions _____

_____

Comments _____

_____

_____

APPOINTMENTS

Date _____

Doctor _____

Location _____

Telephone _____

Questions _____

_____

_____

Comments _____

_____

_____

_____

Date _____

Doctor _____

Location _____

Telephone _____

Questions _____

_____

_____

Comments _____

_____

_____

_____

APPOINTMENTS

Date

Doctor

Location

Telephone

Questions

Comments

Date

Doctor

Location

Telephone

Questions

Comments

RECENT IMPORTANT MEDICAL
RESEARCH PUBLISHED DURING
THE PRINTING OF THIS BOOK

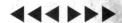

PLEASE DISCUSS THESE RESULTS

WITH YOUR DOCTOR

Prostate Cancer Prevention Should be Tantamount to Heart Disease Prevention

THE FIRST PROSTATE CANCER PREVENTION TRIAL WAS COMPLETED AND THERE WERE SOME ENCOURAGING AND DISCOURAGING RESULTS. DID FINASTERIDE (PROSCAR®) REDUCE THE RISK OF PROSTATE CANCER COMPARED TO A PLACEBO?

The largest chemoprevention trial for prostate cancer recently concluded. This trial was called the "Prostate Cancer Prevention Trial (PCPT)." A total of 18,882 men 55 years of age or older with a normal digital rectal examination (DRE) and a prostate-specific antigen (PSA) level of 3.0 ng/ml or lower were allocated to finasteride (5 mg/d) or placebo for 7 years. In men taking finasteride, prostate cancer was reduced by 24.8% over the 7 years vs. placebo ($P < 0.001$). However, more aggressive prostate cancers (Gleason scores 7–10) were more common in the finasteride group vs. the placebo group ($P < 0.001$). Therefore, finasteride reduced the risk of being diagnosed with prostate cancer, but if you were diagnosed with prostate cancer there was a higher chance of it being more aggressive with finasteride versus placebo. Another way of looking at the numbers is that if 1,000 63-year old men were followed for 7 years, then 60 would get prostate cancer and 18 of the 60 cancers would be more aggressive. However, if 1,000 63-year old men took finasteride for 7 years, only 45 men would get prostate cancer, but 22 of the 60 cancers would be more aggressive. This may sound like a big catch, but researchers have not yet figured out if finasteride actually increases the risk of aggressive prostate cancer, or could this be just a false reading. In other words, some pathologists argue that finasteride gives the appearance of a more aggressive tumor when the tumor itself is not aggressive. Therefore, the pathologists in this study may have classified a prostate cancer in the finasteride group as being more aggressive when it really was not. This answer will not be solved for some time. The researchers from this study are actually doing more intensive research with these tissues to determine whether or not finasteride actually increases the risk of aggressive disease. In the meantime, it is important to know that there were just as many men that died from prostate cancer in the finasteride group versus the placebo group (5 men died of prostate cancer in the finasteride arm and 5 men died from prostate cancer in the placebo arm). In addition, it seems that 1,123 of the approximately 18,882 men died during this 7-year trial (573 or 7% of the men in the finasteride arm and 550 men or 6.7% in the placebo arm died during the study). Most men actually died from cardiovascular disease in this study. Thus, men should be as concerned about their cholesterol levels and other markers for cardiovascular disease as much as they should be concerned about their PSA level. This is also a good lesson from this unique landmark study. Finally, it is also important to mention that sexual-side effects were more common with finasteride, but urinary problems or symptoms were more common in men receiving placebo. Patients should be advised to discuss the latest on-going prevention results with this trial with their current health care provider because more results from this trial will be released in a short period of time (Thompson, I. M.; Goodman, P. J.; Tangen, C. M.; *et al*. The influence of finasteride on the development of prostate cancer. *New England Journal of Medicine* 349:213–222, 2003).

Another large prostate cancer prevention trial that will only include high-risk prostate cancer patients has begun. Patients will receive 0.5 mg of dutasteride (Avodart®) or placebo. Dutasteride has already been approved for non-cancerous enlargement of the prostate or BPH; therefore, discuss this trial with your health care provider. Dutasteride is similar but also a little different than finasteride. However, both drugs tend to reduce your PSA by 50% within 6 months of taking the drug so this has to be corrected for by your physician. Interestingly, dutasteride and finasteride are being tested in patients with prostate cancer to see if they are effective by themselves or along with other prostate cancer treatments, and dutasteride is also being tested as a possible hair growth drug for men with premature baldness. Finasteride was approved for male hair loss several years ago and it is sold under the trade name Propecia® (1 milligram finasteride).

This lower dose of finasteride can also reduce PSA by 50%, so always tell your prostate doctor if you are taking either finasteride or dutasteride.

Looks Like Viagra® (Sildenafil) Has Some Competition Now and in the Future

It turns out that a new pill for erectile dysfunction has now been approved. It is called "Levitra®" *or* "Vardenafil." Talk to your doctor about this and other new drugs and treatments for erectile dysfunction that expect to be available in the future. For example, another pill for erectile dysfunction called "Cialis®" *or* "Tadalafil" may get approved soon as well as a gel or other treatments for this condition. Regardless, please talk with your doctor about the ongoing research for erectile dysfunction because so many exciting drugs or treatments may be available soon. Viagra is a good drug and it will continue to be a good treatment for erectile dysfunction, but patients will have several choices in the next few years and deciding which treatment is best will only occur after an evaluation and discussion with your doctor.

Weight Lifting for Men Receiving Androgen Deprivation Therapy for Prostate Cancer

A total of 155 men with prostate cancer who were scheduled to receive androgen deprivation therapy for at least 3 months were randomly assigned to a weight lifting program 3 times a week for 12 weeks ($n = 82$) or a control group ($n = 73$). Men assigned to weight lifting had less fatigue on activities of daily living ($P = 0.002$) and higher quality of life scores ($P = 0.001$) compared to men in the control group. Men that lifted weights had higher levels of upper body ($P = 0.009$) and lower body ($P < 0.001$) muscular fitness versus men in the control arm. The 12-week weight lifting intervention did not improve body weight, body mass index, waist circumference, or subcutaneous skinfolds. However, lifting weights should be advocated in men receiving androgen deprivation because of the profound impact on fatigue and quality of life (Segal, R. J.; Reid, R. D.; Courneya, K. S.; *et al.* Resistance exercise in men receiving androgen deprivation therapy for prostate cancer. *Journal of Clinical Oncology* 21:1653–1659, 2003).

COX-2 Inhibitors (aka "Super Aspirins") As an Additional Treatment for Prostate Cancer?

Cox-2 inhibitors such as Celebrex®, Vioxx®, and Bextra® (already approved by the FDA for arthritis treatment) are being tested in numerous clinical trials to determine if they can reduce the risk of prostate cancer or have an effect on existing prostate cancer. Our advice is that you ask your doctor on a regular basis about the recent research with COX-2 inhibitors drugs and prostate cancer. We do not know *yet* if they benefit individuals *who have or are hoping to prevent* cancer, but please keep up to date. For example, Celebrex® was recently approved by the FDA for patients at high-risk for colon cancer (a condition called "familial adenomatous polyposis") to reduce polyp formation. It was this study in high-risk colon cancer patients that is part of the reason that there is so much excitement with these drugs for other cancers. Also, keep in mind that *some people believe* daily aspirin may also be an option, *and remember to* check with your doctor first to see if you qualify for aspirin therapy because of a higher risk for cardiovascular disease. Basically, what is heart healthy tends to be prostate healthy, so this should also be remembered. Regardless, aspirin and related compounds along with COX-2 inhibitors could increase your risk of internal bleeding or an ulcer. In addition, researchers are not sure right now whether or not COX-2 inhibitors can protect you from heart disease. Again, talk to your doctor about these issues.

Follow the Ongoing Data with the Anti-osteoporosis Drugs

The oral and I.V. anti-osteoporosis drugs are receiving a lot of attention in cancer research. It seems that they may not only reduce the risk of osteoporosis, but they may also slow the progression of a variety of cancers. Most of these clinical trials have not been concluded, but the research is interesting. For example, the oral drugs such as: Actonel®, Fosamax®, and others may play a role. In addition, the I.V. drugs such as: Aredia®, Zometa®, and others are also being studied. Finally, a drug called "PTH" or Forteo® (daily self-injection) was recently approved for male osteoporosis. There are many potential anti-osteoporosis agents that may have a role in bone health and cancer. Ask your doctor about the latest update on these and other drug therapies. Also, keep in mind that calcium and/or vitamin D supplements should be taken with every anti-osteoporosis drug to enhance the effect of the drug itself.

Fish Oil Supplements or Prescription Vitamin D for Cancer

It is interesting to us that 2003 was the first year that the American Heart Association actually endorses the use of fish oil supplements for patients at high-risk for cardiovascular disease. The recommended dosage is 1 gram per day if your doctor thinks you qualify for this supplement. Fish oil supplements should contain 2 primary compounds called "EPA" and "DHA" and nothing else. These supplements also have been found to have little to no levels of mercury, which is a good thing. Basically, since these supplements are getting so much attention in cardiovascular disease, they are now being studied in prostate cancer. Also, there is a lot of interest in these supplements for patients that have experienced significant weight loss from cancer. It seems that these supplements may also help patients maintain or gain weight in very large supplemental dosages. Again, ask your doctor about the latest research.

Prescription vitamin D (also known as "calcitriol") has been combined with some chemotherapy drugs in an attempt to enhance the effect of the drug itself. For example, one small phase II trial of prescription vitamin D + Taxotere® found that over 80% of the patients with hormone refractory prostate cancer had a PSA response. These results were so encouraging that a large phase III trial at 60 sites is currently being conducted with these 2 agents. Again, ask your doctor about the latest results of these drugs and others for hormone refractory prostate cancer.

New Drug Approved for Benign Prostatic Hyperplasia (BPH)

A new drug called alfuzosin [also known as Uroxatral®] was approved for BPH (non-cancerous enlargement of the prostate). This drug belongs to the class of drugs known as the alpha-blockers, therefore it works by relaxing the prostate. Ask your doctor about the latest results with this and other BPH drugs.